DRUGS TO DISTANT HEALING

My Life-Changing Journey
From Pharmacist to Soul Healer

Veronica Rudan

Co-Authored with Raymond Aaron

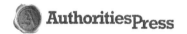

Drugs to Distant Healing: My Life-Changing Journey from Pharmacist to Soul Healer
www.drugstodistanthealing.com

Copyright © 2021 Veronica Rudan

ISBN: 978-1-77277-356-9

Publisher
10-10-10 Publishing
Markham, ON   Canada

Printed in Canada and the United States of America

Table of Contents

To my sister, Milica, whom I love and adore, my heart-felt thanks for always being on my side. Entrusting your healing and life to me with so much grace has led me to where I am today; so without you, I might never have arrived at this point.

With love,
Veronica

Acknowledgements

No woman is an island, and I for one am fortunate to have come across, befriended, loved, and been supported by a community.

I wish to thank **Raymond Aaron,** who encouraged me to be the best version of myself. You instilled in me the confidence to write this book to share my vision with the world.

My gratitude to **Ed Strachar,** my mentor, who threw open the doors to Soul Healing at a time when I was seeking to deepen and widen my healing work. You lead by example and inspire by your willingness to break new ground, while simultaneously enforcing a discipline necessary to high-vibrational healing. You have uplevelled my leadership skills and persuaded me to raise my sights to greater heights.

Thank you to my parents, to whom I owe so much. My father, **Mile,** an exceptional pioneer in his own right, told me to go for whatever I want and to grab it. He encouraged me to think outside the box. My mother, **Irena,** instilled in me the necessary ingredients for success, and the discipline and determination to see to the end whatever it is I embark on.

To my two sons, **Andreas** and **Sascha,** who intuitively know when I need a boost of morale, I thank you for trusting in me, for believing in me, and for supporting the work that I do. Both of you make me smile every day.

My deepest appreciation for my staff at Pharmashield Dispensary in Niagara Falls: **Satyam, Anna, Shawn,** and **Jag;** and drivers, **Wally, Naz,** and **Victor.** I am thankful every day for your dedication and commitment to Pharmashield, and for embodying our heartfelt mission to be of service every day with every client. You are all family, and I couldn't have run the business, nor won accolades from the community, without any of you.

I wish to extend thanks to **Esther Hicks,** whose teachings of Abraham's have inspired me to go higher, further, and faster to achieve my life's purpose in healing. By sharing the valuable teaching that the key is to always have the highest vibration, you have changed my life. Fully understanding that I am what I focus on, and that I am a co-creator with the Divine, has opened immense possibilities and pathways for me.

To **Ridley College,** thank you for providing a fertile environment to nurture forward-thinking, growth and creativity for my kids and other families. It has been a wonderful experience for my children and me, and I see the same for other families, to be given the opportunity to develop an appreciation for arts and sports, and to acquire life skills in public speaking and self -expression. Ridley College is a blessing to the community.

I would like to thank my dear friends **Sarah, Zarina, Tina, Sandra, Kathy** and **Laurie** for always supporting my life decisions and for being towers of strength during those tough times when I questioned myself or my actions. Thank you all for always being there.

There are a few people that have been great teachers to me on my path of expanding my consciousness and my growth as a person.

Marty, thank you for all the lessons I have learned with you. I am grateful for all that you are …you are a unique and one of a kind human being.

My thanks to **Antonio** and **Olivier** for being a part of my life and for co-parenting two beautiful boys.

To my dear friend **Karim,** I deeply appreciate how supportive you are as a friend and how you have my back during my toughest times.

And finally I thank the Divine light of God and all the higher masters that represent love, that have been present with me in all my healings. I am truly and deeply grateful for the love and protection that You have always accorded me.

Foreword

"To everything there is a season, a time for every purpose under heaven." These wise words from Ecclesiastes in the Bible are very apt here. Traditional healing modalities are no longer working and the time has come for soul healing, a breakthrough practice that comes from the new frontiers of energy medicine.

As you may know, you are made of energy. Soul healing deals with the healer downloading very high-level frequencies into your body to bring you back into optimal health and balance. But as author Veronica Rudan describes it, what also makes soul healing so powerful is that it is heart-based, because love is the most powerful frequency in the Universe. While soul healing works immediately and effectively on all forms of dis-ease, maintaining optimal health requires that you love yourself, that you take responsibility for your own health, for letting go of past pain and wounding, and for forgiving, because those are all dense vibrations.

You are in for a treat here, especially if you have been frustrated with what society has accepted as normal: pill popping as the panacea to cover all ills. Be prepared to open your mind and heal your body on a whole new level.

Veronica Rudan has a scientific-based career and profession, but she understands that you are a multi-dimensional being and are, at this stage of your evolution, expanding your awareness of other sacred forms of healing and are willing to accept help from the unseen realms.

In *Drugs to Distant Healing*, you'll discover:

- How soul healing works and why it works
- How it restores the energetic life force that runs through you
- Why it is the modality for this stage of your humanity
- What causes illnesses
- Why the thoughts you think and the words you speak support or hamper your healing
- Easy steps to seal the high level frequencies into your being

Welcome to the Age of Soul Healing!

Loral Langemeier
The Millionaire Maker

1
How It All Started

*"The Soul always knows what to do to heal itself.
The challenge is to quiet the mind."*
– Caroline Myss

One fine Saturday evening in November 2019, I received a text about a miracle that confirmed Soul Healing was absolutely the right path for me. As of this writing, I don't know how the future trajectory of my life will change. But I know that where I am right now, and what I am doing in service to healing others, is exactly where I should be.

The text from a young girl, Mary (her name has been changed for the sake of anonymity), read like this. "…but I wanted to tell you I went to the doctor Thursday, and my holes are starting to fill in with new bone tissue, and I actually keep wondering if it had something to do with the healings you wanted to write about in your book.

"I am not getting an amputation—my doctors are all like wtf. I recorded our conversation…"

Mary, a 20-year-old, had been diagnosed with bone cancer, and her doctors had told her they would need to amputate her left leg from the knee down. I conducted three sessions of Soul Healing on her when she sought out my services as a Soul Healer. In the first session, I cleared her body, energy field, and soul, of negativity, in preparation for the very high frequency Universal Force, which I downloaded into her. During all this time, as I told her, I pictured her as whole and free of cancer, because in the higher realms where Soul Healing takes place, she is perfect.

In the second session, I downloaded high-level frequencies to repair her immune system, her body parts, and organs. In the third and final session, she made peace with dysfunctions in relationships and any past traumas linked to the people in her life that might have played havoc with her emotions.

Each time I worked with Mary, I envisioned her as perfectly whole, and advised her not to talk about the cancer in her leg, nor to dwell on the prospect of amputation, so as not to invite the negative vibrations into her field. To be honest, she was a little sceptical of the process of Soul Healing, but she followed all the steps I recommended to prevent the high-level frequencies from leaking out. Her doctors were astounded by the positive and unexpected reversal in her condition, and they asked her what extra supplements or drugs she was taking, of which there were none. But in her mind, as she told me, she attributed the miraculous recovery to the Soul Healing.

It's been two years since I started Soul Healing while running a pharmacy full time, and I have seen wonderful outcomes. Clients, who had crippling back pains, have stood tall after one or two healing sessions, and those who had severe food allergies were grateful that the allergens no longer bothered them. But Mary's healing is the most astonishing and most breathtaking to date.

I am named Veronica, after my grandmother, Veronika, from Lithuania… But that's not the only thing we have in common. Like my grandma, who was the shaman for the village, I am also a healer, drawing on unseen and unquantifiable realms to channel Soul Healing into the client.

Yes, I am a Soul Healer. And I am also a pharmacist with a popular pharmacy in Niagara Falls, and I see my purpose as not only bridging the worlds of science and the quantum fields in which we are all interconnected, but also in helping clients understand that there is a time and place for different and all forms of healing.

In my practice as a Soul Healer, I recognize that nothing is bad, be it a pharmaceutical prescription or an alternative remedy. It is not a case of all or nothing. It is whatever resonates with the patient. If you were involved in an accident, it's prudent and advisable to get into the emergency. But there are times when an illness or a disease is inexplicable and defies allopathic treatments. That's why Soul Healing is essential, to raise the vibrational frequencies of the client to such a high level so as to restore their healthy blueprint to its original, optimal state, and download remedies of healing into them.

It sounds revolutionary. Clearly, by our conventional standards, Soul Healing stands at the frontier of health and healing. It may be thought of as the future of health care, but

I also support my work with practical tools like exercises, supplements, and managing changes to a client's lifestyle. Soul Healing can be conducted in person, remotely, and over long distances, and it's compatible with all other healing modalities. Unlike in chemical prescriptions, where there may be side effects or contradictions, a Soul Healing has only benefits.

During a Soul Healing, I work with the Divine and higher energetic beings of love and light (you may have a different belief system that acknowledges Buddha or ascended masters), over an average of four sessions. I customize a lifestyle plan and exercises to get my clients to take responsibility for their health. They need to continue the healing work of restoring health and balance in their lives by taking steps to stem energy leaks, which will drain them of the high vibrational frequencies that are now reinvigorating their bodies. This is something I will describe in greater detail further into the book. For now, it is enough to understand that Soul Healing has its roots in Love and Light and in the Heart.

I was introduced to the metaphysical as a very young child, although at that time, I didn't recognize it as such. All I knew was that I had a crippling fear, and my grandmother removed it...with a glass bowl and some incomprehensible words.

Fear of Dogs as a Child

My grandmother first performed a shamanic healing on me when I was a child, to overcome an extreme fear of dogs. When I was five, a large golden retriever jumped on me, and it scared the living daylights out of me. From that point on, when we visited friends who had dogs, they had to corral their dogs into a separate room so that I wouldn't come into contact with them. My fear was so intense that I would start hyperventilating the moment I heard that someone had a dog, even if the dog wasn't anywhere close to me. Just the piece of information that someone I knew had a dog, sent my system into intense panic.

This trauma soon became an issue for my parents because of the fuss and drama everyone had to go through just for a social visit. It also didn't help that most of my parents' friends were dog people.

One day, on a visit to my grandmother, whom I addressed as Babcha, in Montreal, my mother brought up my overwhelming fear. My Babcha was known in her village as a shaman who specialized in curing people of skin disorders and emotional issues, and she would be visited by villagers who could not find appropriate solutions from conventional doctors. She was their healer of last resort.

My Babcha decided to do something to help me, her little Veronica. One morning, I woke up just before dawn at 5 am, and she sat me on a chair. She held a glass bowl over my head, and poured in sacred blessed water with melted beeswax. Then she chanted a strange prayer in words I didn't understand. She repeated the prayer twice, interpreted the formations that the melted beeswax had formed in the bowl, and the ritual was done!

As a kid, I didn't understand what was going on, other than acknowledging that I was very tired and needed to get back into my cozy, warm bed to continue my sleep.

It didn't take long before the efficacy and strength of my grandmother's reputation as a healer was put to the test.

That very afternoon, we paid a visit to my aunt, who had a curly white poodle. On previous occasions, she would take the pains to coop up the dog in a separate room. However, my mom told her sister to leave the dog as it was. It was a test, but one I was fully unaware of.

Putting Healing to the Test

The moment of truth arrived. We rang the doorbell. I walked into my aunt's house, and the poodle sat there, staring at me with his little black eyes. I stared back, not out of anxiety or fear, but out of curiosity. The dog started sniffing out my toes and giving me the smell once-over, like dogs are prone to do. Unlike on previous encounters with dogs, this time, I didn't have a panic attack; I did not hyperventilate, nor did I freak out.

My mom started smiling, and I took the lead from her. A smile slowly formed on my face. It was liberating. I was no longer gripped by harrowing fear, and life could proceed again as normal.

Even though I was still young, I didn't understand how my dread of canines could have been removed with a few words and a ritual with a glass bowl. I could, however, grasp that something miraculous had happened. And that began my journey into unknown and invisible realms, and how they are filled with energies to heal us.

A Journey Into the Unconvential via the Conventional

Looking back with the wisdom I have gained, I recognize fully that my Babcha had performed a shamanistic ritual on me. My mom had informed me that the knowledge of the healer could only be passed down to future generations—verbally, never in writing—to the youngest or oldest child in the family. I am the oldest child.

I took a slightly more conventional path in my education. I went to pharmacy school and, on graduation, had a desire to study naturopathy. I always had an interest in alternative remedies and modalities, and through the years have acquired a storehouse of knowledge and practices, including reiki and reconnective healing. As a fresh graduate, once I discovered that the naturopathy school would require another four years of study, I decided to practice as a pharmacist but continue to delve into the alternative therapies. Intuitively, I knew I wanted to combine the two, and I have done so.

My Babcha's healing of my fright over dogs was my first exposure to her tremendous healing powers. Although her healing genes run in me, mine as a Soul Healer lay dormant for several decades, until I hurt myself with an injury that lasted more than a year. I go into that part of my journey in Chapters 5 and 6.

Soul Healing is Miraculous

Soul Healing is nothing short of miraculous. It can be conducted remotely, over the phone, online, or in person, because in the quantum field, there is no such thing as distance. In the quantum field, we are part of an interconnected web of vibration and frequencies. Healing can happen right away or it may take four sessions, spaced over a period of a month. Some clients may require 5–6 sessions.

I practice Soul Healing on clients with dire diagnoses, or those with a simple case of a bad tummy ache. In fact, I lowered Raymond Aaron's blood pressure by 30 points after one session, and the beneficial effects lasted for several weeks.

There is only a very small group of us Soul Healers in the world. Anything can be healed through Soul Healing. By entering into an altered state of consciousness, I channel the Universal energies, which raises the vibration of a client to a very high level, healing the soul and realigning and enabling the body to heal itself. I am a conduit. I help to elevate the client's vibration, and I introduce these higher-level frequencies into a person by having him or her drink a glass of water that is infused with these frequencies.

Anything can be cured with Soul Healing. It can be chronic Crohn's disease, cancer, a muscle tear, or a back pain. My system of Soul Healing is unique to me and my practice and my body of knowledge. The only area that I avoid is addiction.

I am a single mother of two boys, and both my kids have been healed of their ailments, minor or not, with Soul Healing. My younger son had a speech stutter for many years. After I performed a Soul Healing, it disappeared. However, when he is subject to tremendous stress or suffers a cold, both of which are energy leaks, the stutter returns. I redo the healing process, and I encourage him to keep doing my special exercises.

My fear of dogs left me the moment my Babcha completed her healing ritual. Your body can heal in an instant. I'll share with you how in this book.

2
Prescription Drugs Have a Place in Healing

> *"Healing is a matter of time, but it is sometimes*
> *also a matter of opportunity."*
> **– Hippocrates**

My pharmacy in Niagara Falls is called Pharmacy with a Heart[1] because I believe in heart-based healing. I also subscribe to the premise that there is a connection between the brain and the heart. This link responds to emotions, and the neural signals generated by the variable rhythms of the heart profoundly affects our emotional experience at any moment.

This is the basis of HeartMath® Technology, an innovative approach to managing the heart's intelligence to manage our thoughts and emotions, and in so doing, send harmony and well-being throughout the body.

As a Soul Healer, I recognize that the brain and the heart are two separate sources of intelligence, but aligning these two in an integrated manner is how I approach my healing work. Firstly, I calm the heart and the mind, and when my client is in a state of stillness, Universal energies flow through them, getting the body and the soul to heal themselves.

---

[1] Nominated for a Reader's Choice Award for Best Pharmacy in 2019

Yet I also believe there is a time and space for doctors and conventional medicine for all of us. Conventional or allopathic medicine saves lives, especially when it comes to handling emergencies such as a life-threatening heart attack, a traumatic injury from an accident, a premature birth, or broken bones. There are times when surgery is required, to remove tumours or to stop deadly internal bleeding. There are times when using prescriptions to suppress symptoms are appropriate to facilitate the body's own healing response.

What I am saying is that healing is not an "us versus them" debate. It is not as if when you believe in alternative modalities, you abandon visiting your GP for your regular check-ups. Also, it is not to say that when you are on a regime of blood-pressure pills, you completely ignore stress-reduction modalities such as acupuncture or meditation, or yoga and tai-chi.

All healing approaches have valuable tools, and the best strategy is to use the correct tools available to solve the health problem at hand. An aspirin during an impending heart-attack or a clot-related stroke may buy precious time before help comes, because it acts as an anti-coagulant and thins the blood, thereby preventing a clumping of blood platelets that stop blood flow to the heart.

Conventional medicine has also made significant advances as new technology blooms every day. We now have 3D printed body parts, which can be used for limb and skin replacements, and laparoscopic surgery has removed the need for a surgeon to make cuts measuring up to 6–12 inches long to see what's going on inside a person's body.

Abuse of the System Creates Unhealthy Habits or Addictions

Where it goes wrong is when the patient gets stuck on a vicious cycle of dependence on quick fix prescriptions and surgery. When the patient is over-reliant on the healer—be it a doctor, a surgeon, or an alternative practitioner— and shirks away making lifestyle modifications or simply exercising more, he or she is surrendering all personal responsibility for wellness and healing.

Such a person is trapped in a mind-set that medicine solves all ills, and all that is required is to pop a pill when pain rears its ugly head, and to pop another when the symptoms flare up again. Choices such as diet and lifestyle changes aren't even considered.

That is the beginning of the addiction cycle. We have all heard about the opioid epidemic from the reckless over-prescription of pain opioids. These pills decrease in effectiveness over time but are highly addictive and can easily lead to fatal overdoses. According to *The Globe and Mail*, chronic pain care costs the Canadian economy an estimated $60-billion a year in health care and lost wages and taxes; and over the past three years, 9,000 Canadians have died from opioid overdosing.[2]

---

[2] Kelly, Margo, There's a Chronic Pain Crisis in Canada, and Governments Must Address It, March 29, 2019, https://www.theglobeandmail.com/opinion/article-theres-a-chronic-pain-crisis-in-canada-and-governments-must-address

The numbers are far worse south of the border. An average of 130 Americans die every day from overdosing on opioids, and 70% of all related overdose deaths involve a prescription opioid. You may think that anti-inflammatory drugs like aspirin have little side effects, but if used daily, over the long term, they can cause gastrointestinal complications.

We have become a pill-popping society. Unfortunately, there are other hazards associated with being mindless pill poppers, besides addiction and their other deadly side effects of overuse. Medication, including anxiety drugs such as Diazepam, are showing up in our drinking water because the wastewater plants that catch the nasty bits are not adequately filtering out the pharmaceutical drugs. Wastewater pollution is a growing problem, and everything from beta-blockers for high blood pressure, to birth control pills and contaminants such as lead (in Flint, Michigan), are now in our public water supply.

Balance is Key

It's the general wisdom that allopathic medicine focuses on the disease and its symptoms, and works from the outside in. The healing agent is outside of you. Alternative remedies look at the interconnectedness within the body, and relationships between mind, body, and spirit, and has, as its base premise, that the body is equipped to heal itself once it is given sufficient support.

I believe there is a place for both mindsets. If a pathogen makes its way into a person's body and has progressed significantly, you will need an antibiotic to get rid of it. But there is also a bigger question to consider. Why was the patient's immune system unable to get rid of it? Why is it being compromised, and what is required to rebuild it? Those concerns can best be addressed with a more holistic, alternative approach that may require a combination of detoxing, immune support, acupuncture, or homeopathy. If stress is the main trigger in the patient's life, then in addition to dietary modifications, he or she may need to embark on other stress reduction modalities, such as massage or meditation, for additional support.

I am suggesting that turning away from either practice—conventional or alternative—is to deprive yourself of options. As the patient, you want to make the most informed decision, not settle for what is socially accepted as the right thing to do.

Just as healing modalities are progressing, as humans, we are evolving too. We are becoming more aware of the power of our thoughts to shape our realities, and we are understanding the mind-body-spirit connection in all aspects of our lives. We are moving into the age of energy, and the time has come for Soul Healing to be fully integrated into our lives.

3
The Summer That Changed Everything

> *"The body is a self-healing organism,*
> *so it's really about clearing things out of the way*
> *so the body can heal itself."*
> **– Caroline Myss**

Sometimes in a life, you get a chance to look back to see the different paths you've taken. You reflect on the major intersections you came upon, and how different your life would have been had you taken the right fork, not the left lane at pivotal crossroads in your life. There are some turning points that have such major repercussions that their impact vibrates throughout the rest of your life that is still unlived and yet to unspool.

There was one such turning point for me, and it happened in the summer of 2017. That was the summer that changed EVERYTHING. I couldn't have imagined the twists and turns of the pathway that brought me to Soul Healing, and what I needed to relearn, and the perspectives I had to change.

I was working in my pharmacy, the Pharmacy with a Heart, in Niagara Falls, when an urgent call came through.

"Hello, Veronica here," I answered.

There was a panicked person on the other end, speaking so fast that I could barely make out the words. My sister, Milica, was suffering a psychotic break, was acting really strangely, and was speaking in strange voices. Remember, my grandmother is a shaman from Lithuania, and members of our family had different levels of sensitivity and empathy. It sounded to me that she was having a hard time and was unmoored from reality.

At my store are Color Essence sprays that I had bought from Sedona several years ago. These are water-based sprays infused with light healing properties that vibrationally impact the mind, body, and spirit. The color essences are non-intrusive but bring the person back into equilibrium. We use the color essences either by spraying it on the body or having the person who needs healing drink some water in which some essence is sprayed.

I immediately grabbed the black and opalescent sprays, instructed my delivery driver to leave the sprays at the door of my sister's, and someone inside would open the door to pick it up. They sprayed Black Raven on Milica, had her drink the water, and she fell asleep for four hours. She woke up back to normal with not much of a recollection for what had happened.

I chose Black Raven because it dispels negative energy, and she needed white at night and again in the morning, because the white spray cleanses the auric field and harmonizes the person across all states of being—physical, emotional, and spiritual. So, she went back to normal, but I had little idea that there was more in store for me. I thought that was the end of the excitement for the day.

Oftentimes, I have found that when I am working on Soul Healing, which means I am spreading love and light, something sabotages me. I could be at a meeting, and the systems get disconnected. I could be healing someone, and the lights go out because there are hexes and curses on the person, and we have to persuade or convince the person to let go of the negativity. There will be attempts by negative entities to hijack a healing and I have experienced some of these incidents first hand.

During this particular summer, my sons, who live with me, were 16 and 13 years old. My sister Milica had come to my house earlier that day to ask for help in removing an evil spirit that, according to her, had invaded her home and dragged her down the stairs. I didn't believe her at all, I thought she was once having yet a psychotic break from reality but I said I would hop over to her house after work. She knew I needed to prepare myself with appropriate materials – such as smudges, sage and holy water from Eastern Europe – and I would first pop home after work before driving over to her place. When I walked into my own house intending only to pick up some smudging tools and then immediately turning around for Milica's place, the cabinet doors in my kitchen opened and closed inexplicably on their own, doing so repeatedly for 10 seconds. Eventually, the situation returned to normal, and everything was as if nothing had happened, but that incident is permanently seared in my mind. Looking back now, it was as if Milica had brought some of the evil over when she came to my home in the afternoon and it turned on the scare tactics to stop me from smudging her place to get rid of the spirit attachment. I have a scientific background and if you had told me this would happen to anyone let alone me, I would have pooh-poohed it and laughed it off. As it was, my sons and I stood in the kitchen confounded and while we really didn't understand then what was going on, we stood firm and didn't give in to the fear.

That was the moment I came so close to a realm outside our normal three-dimensional (3D) reality. That was my first close brush with the supernatural. I am not talking about some mumbo-jumbo; I am a pragmatic grounded person, but the more I delve into levels of healing, the more I recognize that there are different realms beyond our existence. Perhaps it may help if we look at a definition of the word *supernatural*. The Oxford English Dictionary defines the adjective as follows:

su·per·nat·u·ral: (of a manifestation or event) attributed to some force beyond scientific understanding or the laws of nature.

A supernatural event is something outside of our immediate understanding, but just because we don't see it doesn't mean it doesn't exist. The incidents of that particular day that summer taught me a lesson and gave me a new perspective. It was my lightbulb moment. Evil does exist; evil in the form of curses and hexes can affect a person's health, and healing systems in this Age of Energy have to take that into account

It may sound far-fetched, but in our 3D realities, we've always grasped in different cultural traditions some concept of clearing the energies of the home. These cultures believe that the energy of a person you come into contact with, whether the person's vibes are positive or negative, tend to linger in your field; likewise with the home.

If the energies in a particular home are stressful and confrontational, those energies will gather like dust balls, and will need to be cleared out. First Nation and the Native American tribes smudge with leafy bundles of sage or smudge sticks to cleanse a space and rid it of heavy, dark energies, leaving behind an airy, peaceful, restful home. They believe the life force energy of the sage flows into the ether and changes the vibration of a space or person, by absorbing dense energy and impurities. As an aside, it has been shown in scientific journals that medicinal smoke from sage would clear 94% of airborne bacteria in the air in a confined space.[3]

In the Chinese Feng Shui tradition, cleansing is done with any number of tools, including bells to create cleansing frequencies and to raise the vibrational level of a space. In other Eastern belief systems, such as Buddhism and Shintoism, salt is used to repel evil and to cleanse.

Soul Healing does all this and more, without having to stock up on this cleansing tool or another, or carry bells or crystals

---

[3] Nautiyal CS1, Chauhan PS, Nene YL, Medicinal smoke reduces airborne bacteria, J Ethnopharmacol. 2007 Dec 3;114(3):446-51. Epub 2007 Aug 28

or colour essences. Such things are good to have, and some people are more comfortable being able to feel a physical object, but Soul Healing transcends the physical dimension.

Downloading Informatioinal Remedies

We are all multi-dimensional beings, and we are waking up. We are moving from our narrowly focused and limited 3D reality into the elevated vibrations of the higher dimensions. We are awakening to our greatness within, and we need new ways of healing in the higher dimension. Only a form of healing that embodies mind, body, and spirit can work. In my Soul Healing, I shift energetic patterns to usher in physical healing at the cellular level, greater joy, and happiness.

I had delved very deeply into various healing modalities, like homeopathy, before I met Ed Strachar, who launched me into the world of Soul Healing. One such teacher, whom I am very grateful for, is Catherine Bradley, who introduced me to Heilkunst Homeopathy, which amongst other things, uses dynamic or energetic remedies to heal. However, the one remarkable thing I learned from Catherine is that we can download the essence of a homeopathic remedy, without needing the physical capsules to facilitate a cure.

Not too long ago, I was on the phone with a writer friend of mine who was suffering severely from allergies. She was in a bit of physical distress, and because she couldn't mute the conversation in time, she sneezed loudly into the micro-phone, almost blowing up my eardrum! She was very apologetic about it, and explained that she was a big user of homeopathic remedies but had run out of the Histaminum that she normally used to control her allergies.

She was actually starting to stress out about not having her regular supplies on hand, because her allergies were very troubling. Once she got them, she would be extremely tired, be coughing incessantly, suffer a runny nose, and the skin around her upper lip and nose would be rubbed raw from her having to use copious sheets of tissue paper.

I immediately suggested to her to use Allium Cepa, a homeopathic remedy made from onions, but rather than waiting till she could get off the phone and run to the store to get the capsules, I told her to write the words *Allium Cepa 200C* (this indicates the level of dilution; see Appendix for more on homeopathy) on her arm. She didn't have a marker nearby, so she just went through the motions of scribbling the remedy name and the dilution, with her finger, on her arm, and she felt better almost immediately. She has since happily relied on this method of "writing" on her arm to help with little health issues.

She recently told me that she used the same technique for a bee sting. Most people stung by a bee can experience severe burning pain at the site of the sting, for several hours, while the swelling from the venom can increase and last for any length of time, from two to seven hours.

My friend's experience was very different, thankfully. She was sitting by a swimming pool and, strangely enough, there were bees swarming around her. Without her knowing it, a bee had landed on her sandal, and as she stood up to get away from the bees, the one in her sandal stung her and buried the stinger in the arch of her foot. Gingerly, she removed the stinger from her foot and was upset because she was on a short holiday. Now everything was going to be messed up. She was in pain when she jumped into the pool to wash off any scent or fragrance that might have attracted the bees.

Then she remembered my suggestion, so she asked her husband to google homeopathics for bee stings. He came up with Apis Mellifica, and she immediately stopped swimming, and "wrote" down Apis Mellifica 6C on her foot. She felt the pain decreasing, and repeated the same thing 5 minutes later. In homeopathy, if you use a low dilution, frequency of use is the key. To cut a story short, the pain disappeared, and she had no swelling or pain; neither was there a welt on her foot.

I call this method an informational remedy; it works because we download the energy or essence, or in other words, the information of the cure into our bodies. I have used it on myself and written names of homeopathic cures on my arm to reduce anxiety. I would notice the difference in 10–15 minutes. I also pen words like *peace, calm,* and *love,* on pieces of paper, which I scatter throughout my house to keep it vibrating at an elevated level.

These days, this kind of vibrational healing is commonplace to me, but I can still remember vividly the first time I handled a healing this way. The pharmaceutical technician in my workplace suddenly suffered from severe hiccups. I was conducting a Soul Healing on her to alleviate her anxiety, and she suddenly started hiccupping non-stop. I knew that the remedy Magnesium Phosphorica 6X would help her.

I realized I didn't have it in the store but figured out I could download the essence of the energy into her. As she was still energetically open from the Soul Healing, I thought it would work. The hiccups stopped immediately, to her surprise and relief! I wouldn't have believed that this kind of informational remedy would work so effectively or as speedily as it did, had I not seen it with my own eyes. But now I no longer question the effectiveness of energy healing.

This kind of healing works very well with animals too. One of my dogs got a bad cut from running through the woods. Rather than further stressing him out by taking him to the vet and feeding prescriptions to him orally, I aligned with the Universe and downloaded a healing into him. I did it by downloading water from the purest lake in the world, mixing it with some homeopathic remedies four times a day, and he became calmer, which was a prerequisite to his healing.

Informational cures are just one aspect of Soul Healing. I work on the quantum field when I am conducting a Soul Healing, the field where we are all interconnected. Before downloading any remedies to a client, my kids, or myself, I send love to the spirit of the remedy. Then I download it, a process which takes seconds, and I give thanks from my heart. All Soul Healing is heart-based because the heart is an important carrier of information. According to the Heart Math Institute (HMI), the magnetic field around the heart envelops every cell in our bodies and reaches out several feet around us. It's also 100 times greater than the field created by the brain. Just as importantly, heart-based means love-based, and love conquers all obstacles, and overcomes all barriers.

This kind of informational remedy is just one aspect of Soul Healing. It is quite similar to the discoveries by Dr. Masaru Emoto, who showed that prayers, thoughts, and words influence water by showing the before and after crystalline patterns in water. Positive uplifting words, like *love, thank you,* and *you are beautiful,* create beautiful water crystals, while negative, angry, and depressing words led to badly bent and deformed crystalline patterns. If simple words can affect water molecules, how much more would they affect us, since our bodies are 70% water?

In subsequent chapters, I will go into further detail of how Soul Healing works. But let me add here that Soul Healing works miraculously, but it's also up to the patient to commit to taking maintenance steps to make sure he or she remains at a high vibrational level.

Life happens, and if they fall back into emotional states of stress and anger, they suffer energy leaks, and the ailment that they were healed from may return. When you undergo a Soul Healing, you have to be committed to sustaining your good health by keeping your vibration high. In other words, you have to raise your level of awareness and consciousness to match the higher vibrations that have been downloaded into your body.

Like attracts like, and the elevated healing vibrations will stay if the patient is operating at higher frequencies by putting positive energies into their words, eating good food, and focusing on positive thoughts. It does take the body some days to process the newer light frequencies, and I like to space my sessions for Soul Healing a week or a couple of weeks apart.

Why settle for older, outmoded forms of healing when we are changing dimensionally? There is a new wisdom to tap into, and it's the wisdom of our Soul.

4
Meeting Ed Strachar, Discovering Soul Healing

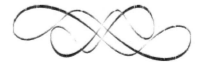

"If it lowers your vibration, it's not for you.
That's how you'll know."
– Lalah Delia

Have you longed to stop going through the motions of life, and find purpose that fires you up? Have you felt that there are missing pieces in your life, and you are unsure as to how to go about making your life whole again?

The Universe is always ready to answer you and give you guidance, but sometimes the message comes in the form of a roadblock. I was looking to get off the conventional path, but it took a twisted ankle, in my case, to set out on a totally different journey to becoming a world-class Soul Healer.

I was out geocaching with my two boys. Geocaching is like an outdoor treasure hunt, in which you use a GPS or other navigational aids on a mobile device to get you to specific locations where containers or geocaches are hidden by other players. Once you find these geocaches, you log in your findings on the internet, and you replace the item you found with something else.

There are different types of caches: physical items such as logbooks, pencils, or items that can be traded with other players. There is also an earth cache, which highlights the natural features of a particular area, such as a historic site or a marine conservation area. Sizes of caches range from micro to multi caches, which are hidden in several locations, or mystery caches that involve coming up with solutions to a puzzle. It's a fun way of exploring the outdoors.

We were pretty caught up in the game and had to go down a hill. On the descent, I slipped and twisted my left ankle. I did everything I knew to heal the injury. By that time, I had spent 10 years studying different alternative modalities, from reiki to homeopathy to connective tissue therapy. I had massage, and went through physiotherapy and laser therapy, but nothing healed the ankle. Even my Core Inergetix machine, which is a technology that scans a person's energy field for points of imbalance, and corrects and resets to restore natural balance, didn't fix the issue.

I had to live with a painful ankle for 1.5 years, and had to wear a brace daily. Soon after the summer of the pivotal moment when the kitchen cabinet doors mysteriously opened on their own accord, I happened to see a Facebook post by a man called Ed Strachar. He mentioned dark energies and offered a healing podcast for a small amount of money. I was intrigued and was willing to join in the podcast since I wasn't risking a whole lot of money. This was my first experience with him.

On the day of the podcast, I had a glass of water next to the computer, as instructed. I turned on the computer, had it on speaker, and signed on to the podcast with 200 other people. It lasted for almost an hour. Then I drank the water in the glass, which had been energized by the healing. I noticed that after the healing, the pain in my ankle was reduced. If it had been at a 10 when I started listening to the podcast, the level of pain had dropped down to a 6. Hours later, I felt that the pain I had lived with for 18 months had almost completely disappeared. Pain had dropped to a 2 on a scale of 1–10.

The jury was still out that day as to how effective the remote healing was, and it wasn't just targeted at me. Hundreds of people from all over the world had logged in. The next day, my ankle still felt good and strong. I decided not to wear the brace that day and, over the day, it improved even more, till it was back to normal.

I was fully intrigued with his method of healing, and was keen to know more. During the podcast, Ed had mentioned that he would be teaching a week-long seminar to a small group of people in Sedona, Arizona. The only bug was that it came with a hefty price tag of US$30,000, including accommodation and food. I didn't have that amount of money on me. In Canadian dollars, the cost worked out to $40,000, which is the annual salary for a fresh graduate here. As a single mother of two, I was mindful of how I spent my money. Nonetheless, I was very keen to go, so I said to myself, "I don't know how I am going to get to the seminar. But I know that I am." I put out the intention to the Universe, and forgot about it.

It was in November then, and the seminar was a month away, in December. I didn't give it another thought, nor did I agonize over how I was going to raise the required funds.

I had put out my desire to the Universe, and I had no expectations as to how the Universe would answer me.

About 10 days after the podcast, my mom asked me about my ankle, having noticed that I was no longer hobbling around with an ankle brace. I described the podcast and how my ankle became normal again soon after, and I also told her about the class. I was very enthusiastic about enrolling in his Healing Genius Mastery Course to draw on Universal energy, because I would be able to help others heal themselves of anything, I told her.

Yes, I am a pharmacist with a scientific background, but I had always intuitively wanted to merge the two, allopathic and alternative, to get the best healing results. I was very influenced by and very connected to my grandmother who is a shaman healer.

She was very passionate about helping others, and she worked very hard for her family and her patients. Although she only had a Grade 3 education and worked in the mines, she also ran a fabric business out of the basement in her home, and successfully bought and flipped properties. She was such a savvy property investor that she gifted each of her five daughters a house, fully paid. I feel so close to my grandmother that I sometimes think I have inherited the healing DNA from her.

Miracles do happen, and one happened to me barely two weeks away from the seminar date. My mom told my extended family about my desire to study with Ed Strachar, and they got together and pooled their money. I felt so blessed by their kindness, and I was grateful that the Universe had manifested my deep soul desire.

At the same time, I felt I had been specially chosen to be bestowed ancient knowledge. The healer gene from my grandmother already ran in my veins, and the financial gift from my family would help me upraise my healing skills to an elevated level. My family understood that health is crucial to an abundant life; without balanced health, we are unable to achieve happiness and financial freedom, and we are not in any position to give something back to the community and the world.

In Arizona, seven of us got together, 10 hours a day, in Ed's workshop. He taught us to open ourselves so that we could tap into Universal energy, and to heal with very high vibrational frequencies. We are part of a very small select group of Soul Healers in the world, who are able to download such powerful vibrations to restore balance and optimal health to those in need. At the same time, our work seeks to empower others to heal themselves.

There were many powerful principles that I learned in the seminar, and among them were how to:

- Connect to the higher dimensions in the Universal energy fields and Mother Earth.
- Transform energy. Energy cannot be eradicated, but it can be transformed.

* Clean negative memories, trauma, emotions and disappointments.
• Protect the soul from negative events.
• Energetically shield myself as a healer, cleaning my own energy field every day to reinvigorate the body and soul.

Those of us who have studied with Ed still get together once a month to share case studies and exchange notes. We are part of a unique community in which we support each other as we carry out this very special, high-vibrational work.

My Own Healing System

I follow a four-step healing system that has achieved wonders. I call it Soul Healing. I am able to see a person's vibrational field and the strength of his or her soul. The more I delve into Soul Healing, the more intuitive I become. Sometimes I see dark energies in a person's field, brought about by cutting words that become a curse that manifests in a person's body as an illness. Yes, illnesses can be caused by hexes, curses, and negative spirits.

Soul Healing is miraculous, but I encourage my patients to not regard it as a pill that they can pop to cure all ills. It is an energy modality that requires patients to commit to their own self-care after each healing session. It's a commitment that will make or break their health. The high-level frequencies that have been downloaded into them will diminish in potency or leak away completely if they don't stick to a prescribed programme of maintenance, which includes clearing their energies daily. For example, when I have some alcohol, some of my ankle pain returns.

Here is a fun aside: Alcohol was previously commonly referred to as "spirits," because it makes the body more vulnerable to negative spirits, and lowers the immune system's resistance to disease.

I am, however, well placed in a position to reboot my body, to clear my body's vibration to re-energize the liver so that it can remove the toxins and the negativity. However, my patients have to recognize that their illnesses will return if they go back to their old ways.

An energy leak isn't just caused by inappropriate foods. It can be created just by a downshift in our thoughts, if we allow negative emotions to flood our bodies. One of my sons has a speech stutter. After I conducted a Soul Healing on him, the stutter disappeared. But when he is stressed, thereby forming an energy leak, the stutter returns. As he is my son, I redo the healing and encourage him to do the energy clearing exercises.

Incidentally, I have included a free energy clearing exercise that can be easily downloaded at my website, drugstodistant healing.com.

You can transform anything through energy healing—any intolerance or allergy, body mechanical issues like back pain or knee pain, and auto-immune and life-threatening diseases, including even cancer.

In the case of patients whose illnesses or emotional imbalances are triggered by trauma with parents or family, Soul Healing will only achieve limited results if they can't bring themselves to forgive whoever they felt had wounded them. By staying in victim mode, they create leaks through which the high-level frequencies will leave their bodies.

However, if they shift their perspective and forgive those who had caused them pain, without judgement or anger, they will be able to shed their previous illnesses or disorders. They can do that by reframing their past pain as a lesson for the soul, and that the people who were instruments of the pain were specifically in the patient's life for that important lesson. Healing at the level of the soul doesn't take place by changing the external circumstances. It happens when you change how you react to the same circumstances.

And if you goof up, don't be so hard on yourself. Self-criticism will easily hit you like a runaway train and derail your progress. Instead, think that you reboot every morning and every night.

Every night, you've the opportunity to clear yourself of any negativity that may have worked its way into your energy field, and to forgive those who may have angered you. Every morning, you have the potential to create a brand-new day, rich in amazing promise and potential.

Who is Ed Strachar?

Ed is a multi-faceted, multi-talented man who is a gifted remote distance healer—a healing teacher who has taught in 50 countries. He has been a mathematician and engineer, author, and speaker. Yet at one stage in his life, Ed was flat broke, downright depressed, and ready to take his own life. Before he bit the bullet, he heard about a vibrational healer and dowser named Raymon Grace, and set up a healing session with him.

Raymon found that Ed was carrying around very heavy negativities, and he told Ed to wait 24 hours for the healing benefits to manifest. As Ed tells it, he felt great the next day. He was no longer weighed down by depression; on the contrary, he felt as if a huge burden had been lifted. Life looked brighter, and suicide was no longer on the menu.

If you look at Ed's condition from a physiological point of view, he could have been suffering from a severe imbalance of chemicals in the brain, and Raymon's healing corrected the unhealthy disparity. So startled and inspired by this amazing turnaround in his life, Ed managed to find some money to drive from Daytona Beach, where he was living, to attend Raymon's seminar. He hasn't looked back since. He has built on his mentor's teachings and is empowering people to heal.

We are in the Age of Energy

Soul Healing may sound far-fetched to the conventional minded. But as I have previously mentioned, we are in the Age of Energy. We are in an extraordinary time when we can learn how to empower ourselves to tap our fullest human potential. The Universe is made of energy; we are made of energy. We are much more than physical matter and bones and sinew. We are emotions, we are thought, and we are spirit. Soul Healing draws on the Life Force that is all around us, to restore our entire being — the body, mind, and spirit — to a state of wellness, freedom, and abundance.

We are much more than what we appear to be. Don't let fear and the conventions of the world box you into what no longer works.

It was *New York Times* best-selling author, Dodinksy, who said, "The key to being happy is knowing you have the power to choose what to accept and what to let go."

Soul Healing appears far-fetched to many who are wedded to science and conventional medicine, and who find it so far outside their comfort zone and zone of belief, that they dismiss it or ignore it outright. But the good news is that you don't have to believe in it. You just have to jump into it, and let the high energies in.

The time for Soul Healing has come.

5
Healing with Higher Vibrational Frequencies

> *"Complete health and awakening*
> *are really the same."*
> **– Tarthang Tulka**

Distance doesn't matter when it comes to Soul Healing. You can be sitting next to me, be sick in bed halfway across town, or standing thousands of miles away in a different time zone. I can be healing one person or a hundred. Like Ed Strachar did with me, I can heal 100 people through a podcast. In Soul Healing, we work with energy and download very high vibrational frequencies into the person, so distance and proximity are not of consequence.

Many people will reject this claim outright, without further thought, because something unseen, like energy as a modality of healing, is too far-fetched. But we are entering a time when we realize we've rejected our own immense potential as humans, and lived very narrow and limited lives. There are many people who surrender their power to institutions and the opinions of others, and who believe that healing is only possible through pharmaceuticals, chemical treatments, and surgery. They believe what they have been told, and have depressed their own ability to discern what truth is, and denied the voice of their inner wisdom.

Let's take a pause here. You cannot see electricity, yet it powers your car, your computer, your mobile devices, and lights up your highways. There are days when you feel so good, you can conquer mountains, and there are moments when you can barely lift a finger. When there is energy coursing through your body, everything seems possible, even moving mountains.

Yet when the life force energy is diminished, life seems harder and more difficult to manage. You are greatly impacted by the differentials in your energy, which you cannot see or touch. You can only feel its power. So, why can't you be healed by energy? You can. I was, my clients have been, and so can you, if you open your mind to explore possibilities beyond what you know and what you have been told.

I am writing this book to invite you to explore this miraculous modality for optimal health and wellbeing. It has no negative side effects, and it places you in a place of empowerment to play a significant role in healing yourself. You don't have to take a lifetime's worth of drugs or supplements, and you'll see substantial benefits after one session.

Soul Healing cures any form of illness, whether it be:

- Physical imbalances, such as back pain, headaches, allergies, chronic fatigue, and insomnia.
- Emotional imbalances, including anxiety, depression, anger, and feeling disconnected.
- Spiritual imbalances for illnesses brought on by evil spirits, demons, hexes, curses, negative spirit guides, or negative soul contracts.

My 4-Step Soul Healing Process

I use a four-step Soul Healing process:

Step 1:

The first stage is a consult to see what is ailing the patient. It is also extremely important for the client to understand that he or she must enter into the healing session without any expectation of being restored to full health.

I cannot stress how important it is to enter the healing session with that clarity. The expectation of being healed is in itself a mental block; it is a white noise that disrupts the universal healing forces. It prejudges and anticipates what shape the healing should take, inadvertently creating a form of resistance to the life force that is to be downloaded.

Clinging to this expectation means the person is stuck in his mind, rather than moving his consciousness to his heart. It's important to let go of attachment for the energy to flow better, and to shift from head to heart, because all transformational soul-based healing come from love—from the Divine and the Universe.

Next, I enter into a meditative state to still my mind, to clear it. I connect to Source, I expand my heart consciousness, and I open up my spiritual channel to see what negativities are ailing the client.

I get the client into a relaxed state, because if a person is all strung up or coiled up in tension, the life force won't flow smoothly. I walk the person through some breathing exercises to still the mind, and guide him or her through a guided visualization to get to a point of stillness and heart-centredness. I also reach out intuitively to check the client's mental resistance, to see if the person is in a sufficiently open state to receive the high-level frequencies.

Then I proceed with clearing and energising the healing space by calling on powerful high-level beings and healing guides, such as angels and saints (you can choose any divine spirit that is meaningful to you).

Next, I clear the energy field around the client, and remove any negativities in the client, to raise the person's frequency to be aligned with optimal health, and to fully receive the healing life force.

Once that is done, I download the Universal life force into the client, acting as a conduit for healing energies that will refresh and renew the client's vibrational field. The work completed at this stage is sufficient to get many clients back on their feet. Some don't come back for a second session, although those with more debilitating conditions will need to do so.

In my world as a pharmacist, I am in constant contact with pharmaceutical sales representatives. One of them, whom I had known for a long time, had missed an appointment. He called to say he was so sick he couldn't lift his head off his pillow. He asked me for a healing over the phone, which I did, and he felt much better; in fact, he felt good enough to get out of his bed and go to work.

I once received a phone call at midnight from the mother of one of my son's classmates. Her son, Quinn, had been sick for three days with the stomach flu. She asked me what I could do to help. My pharmacist training kicked in, and I recommended lots of fluids, and Gravol to stop the nausea.

She replied, "No, Veronica; I want you to do a healing on him."

"Now?" I asked.

"Yes, now," she replied.

I asked to call back in 10 minutes and had them set up a glass of water by Quinn's bedside. I called him and conducted the healing process over the phone. I brought him into the state of stillness that would ensure that he would be most receptive to the healing energies, and the healing was finished 35–40 minutes later.

I had him drink the glass of water, and Quinn said he felt so much better; in fact, he felt great. His level of pain and discomfort had fallen from an 8 (which was the number he picked to indicate his state of illness before we started) to a 3.

The next day, he felt good enough to go back to school. Kids can be sceptical of anything that seems far-fetched to them, but it appeared that Quinn was convinced by his recovery. At school, he told my son, Sascha, that he was a lucky boy because his mom could help realign people so that they can heal themselves, and so quickly too!!

These two cases show that Soul Healing can be immediately effective. You don't have to be going back for repeat sessions, which you may have to for therapies such as massage, reiki, osteopathy, detoxing programmes, or nutritional supplements. Your body can be restored to full health in a single session, and the benefits will stay as long as you take the recommended steps and exercises to avoid energy leaks, which would drain the high-level energy from your body.

It also takes the body a few days to process the changes, and I usually follow up with a call. Sometimes it is sufficient just to have a chat, rather than a repeat of the healing.

In the case of my patient, Dragica B, with whom I am working, she showed noticeable improvement after her first Soul Healing session. Diagnosed with Stage 4 cancer, she felt less pain in her legs, and gained more energy after our first session together.

As it stands, her diagnosis was Stage 4 cancer, but the week after her first healing with me, the doctors revised their opinion to Stage 3 cancer. They said they must have made a mistake the first time around, which is an awful state of affairs; and maybe it was just a coincidence that they downgraded the prognosis, but in the field of energy medicine, things can move very quickly. However, I know, and my patient knows, deep down in her heart, that it was the Soul Healing that significantly improved her condition. Since then, she has been following all the exercises I have shown her; she is suffering noticeably reduced pain, and she has become more positive about her healing journey.

Step 2:

In this step, I get in touch with the spirits of the organs to reinvigorate the body. Everything has a spirit. Plants and trees have spirits, water does, and remedies do. When I download homeopathic remedies into my clients, I am downloading the spirit of the remedy.

As part of Soul Healing, I communicate with the soul and consciousness of the body, the nervous systems, organs, and cells to ask them to heal themselves and to replenish and renew the body. To heal, I call on the high-level guides and beings to work on and reset the cellular structure of the body.

For example, cancer thrives on an acidic environment in the body. I strengthen the spirit of the liver with Divine Energy, to get it to properly detoxify the body in order to restore an alkaline environment, in which the cells can rejuvenate and replenish.

There are 75 trillion cells in each of our bodies, all of which are working in delicate balance to get us to breathe, get up, walk, run, work, imagine, create, live, play, and rest. Stress disrupts the hormonal balances that help these cells do their work, and shortens the telomeres that protect our cells, leading to premature cellular aging and death.

The Divine Energy recharges the cells and gets them to vibrate actively. In the relatively new field of cell seismology, it is shown that elasticity is fundamental to healthy cells. Cancerous cells have corrupted internal machinery, and they become rigid, and conditions such as atherosclerosis and vascular aneurysms begin with a loss of elasticity in the cells and arteries.[4] That is why Soul Healing is so simply effective, because vibrations and frequencies work at the most basic level of life, and retune them to optimal performance.

One of my clients, Carlos, suffered an injury that led to a broken tailbone. His work required that he be on the road constantly, but because of his fracture, he couldn't sit for any length of time in a car. Sitting in a car seat for hours created too much pressure on his tailbone, causing excruciating pain. He was at his wit's end when he approached me for a Soul Healing.

By the second treatment, he was feeling significantly better. In fact, he felt so good, he proceeded to a birthday party. I had advised him against drinking, as alcohol would cancel the benefits of the healing. Unfortunately, he ignored or forgot my recommendation, and when I spoke to him the following week, he complained that the soreness had returned to his back.

---

[4] Cellular seismology: Putting vibrations on the map, University of Montreal Hospital Research Centre (CRCHUM), January 16, 2018, Science Daily, https://www.sciencedaily.com/releases/2018/01/180116111124.htm

I repeated the second treatment to get him feeling better, and this time he avoided alcohol, so as not to suffer a relapse.

Another client, whom I shall call Neil B, suffered from chronic diarrhoea. The doctors couldn't figure out the cause, and the end result was that he couldn't leave the house; neither could he hold on to a job. He needed quick and easy access to the bathroom, and because he couldn't keep nutrients in his body and was constantly dehydrated, he lost 100 pounds.

He went through two sessions of Soul Healing. But in between the first and second stages of my process, he diligently carried out my recommended exercises twice a day. A week later, after giving the body time to adjust to clearing it of negativities, we proceeded with the second stage, after which he felt that he was returning to normal.

Step 3:

Healing is interwoven with how a person lives his or her life. At this stage, I clear the energetics of relationships and any negativities arising from damaging relationships that don't support or nourish, but instead drain and deplete. A person can be stuck in a trauma from an abusive childhood, a co-dependent relationship, or a detrimental work environment. Such people are unable to free themselves from the unconscious emotions that the trauma generates, and which keeps them trapped in the same dense field.

Soul Healing will help a client adopt positive thoughts, feelings, and beliefs that support recovery, but if a person insists on replaying or reliving the memories of trauma, the benefits are diminished.

Step 4:

I redo everything that has been done before. I reinstate healing energies, and revisit any aspects that may require rebalancing, or reinforce those areas that may have been affected by energy leaks. At this stage, if a person shows resistance to healing, I use special techniques to identify any subconscious beliefs that hijack the results of Soul Healing.

I should add that the exercises I recommend should be carried out every day to ensure successful healing. Think of it like brushing your teeth. You don't just brush them once and be done with it. You need to do it at least once a day, and often twice, to keep them clean and free of bacteria. Energy works the same way. You need to maintain the exercises daily to solidify your healing progress.

Group Healing

Once, I was invited to do a presentation on pharmaceuticals in a senior residents' home. The talk was about appropriate level of prescriptions and vitamins, and how to clean up your cabinet of expired and unnecessary medications. The activities director was open to my suggestion to conduct a group healing on the seniors, most of whom were just nodding off on their chairs. They didn't seem engaged in any activity of conversation, and were just keeping to themselves.

I carried out a special healing on them, and the activities director was delighted with the results. She later told me that there was a pool table in the activities room, which had been left unused because no one showed any interest in having a game. However, after the Soul Healing, she noticed that three of the older gentlemen got up to play a game with each other! They felt strong enough and mobile enough to rally together for a game. That was wonderful news. It was assuring to hear that the seniors were benefitting from the recharged energy flowing into and through their bodies, so much so that they felt strong enough to get off their chairs to play a game together.

The Full Package

Healing doesn't have to be difficult. In fact, healing should be and can be very simple.

There are, however, occasions when I support my healing sessions with the Core Inergetix Quantum machine. The quantum machine is totally non-invasive and is designed to accurately detect changes in the quantum frequencies of the cells, and to infuse the body with quantum waves to revert the body's frequencies to their optimal states. This particular machine has 1000 healing modalities to restore health to a person.

I enter the client's pertinent information into the machine, including such details as the place of birth, birthday, and a photo.

The machine conducts a scan, looks at every cell, tissue, and organ of the body, and compares it to a library of optimal frequencies to determine what the stressors are in the body, and comes up with remedies.

I look at the Core Inergetix Quantum machine as a supplemental healing tool, and to offer an alternative to those people who may be sceptical of Soul Healing itself. It is also capable of long-distance healing, as I have successfully used it on clients from as far away as Australia.

There are many people who have been groomed to believe that the body is just a mechanical vehicle that will inevitably run down from years of use. They ignore the mind-body-spirit connection, and do not believe that their emotions, beliefs, and mind-set have as much impact on their health as what they eat and do.

These clients may find it harder to suspend their disbelief of energy work, and will need additional support. For such groups of people, I also provide coaching on healthy habits, from nutrition to meditation, health enhancing supplements, and appropriate energy clearing exercises. You can download a free exercise to clear your energy field, from my website, **drugstodistanthealing.com**. It's easy to do, and it keeps your field clear of leaks that drain you of the life force.

You may be dealing with a health challenge or are just looking to optimise your health. You may be just starting your healing journey or are desperate for solutions because of a chronic disease. Be comforted by the fact that there is a positive health revolution happening, and Soul Healing is right at the forefront of this wave.

Good health and all that comes with it is part of your birthright, but in this day and age of spiralling medical costs, long lines at emergency, and insufficient medical and nursing staff, getting the right kind of care seems like a long haul. Then too, you may have to bounce from one doctor to another to get the proper diagnosis and the support that you need.

Soul Healing may seem radical, but it is authentic, it is powerful, and it is time-saving. It appears simple, but it produces profound results so that you can get on with your life.

6
Steps of the Healing

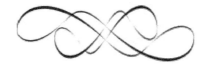

"Our bodies ultimately are fields of information, intelligence, and energy. Quantum healing involves a shift in the fields of energy information, so as to bring about a correction in an idea that has gone wrong."
– Deepak Chopra

We don't live in a vacuum. We have families, friends, and colleagues. We live in cities or towns or the country, and we have dreams, desires, and disappointments. We get frustrated when life doesn't quite pan out the way we had expected, and sometimes we get a blow so hard that we withdraw into ourselves. And other times, life serves us a big, wonderful surprise, like when we fall in love. Whatever it is, as humans, we go through a variety of experiences. A hundred of us could go through the same experience, and we would have a 100 different reactions and responses.

Some of us bounce back like a rubber ball from setbacks, all ready to try it again. For these people, failure is an inconvenience, not a defeat. Others get so invested in the notion that they have to succeed every time that a simple obstacle becomes a huge setback. And they get severely disappointed; the sense of failure seeps into their bodies and throws the bio-chemicals out of whack. Eventually, the emotional blocks manifest as a dis-ease somewhere in the body.

It was Dr. Bruce H. Lipton, stem cell biologist, and bestselling author of *The Biology of Belief,* who pointed out that "Biological behaviour can be controlled by invisible forces, including thought, as well as it can be controlled by physical molecules like penicillin, a fact that provides the scientific underpinning for pharmaceutical-free energy medicine."

You have to recognize that your body is not a machine that runs down from years of use, and healing is not just a question of tinkering with the parts to get the vehicle running again. Your body is not just a miraculous collection of skin, tissue, organs, and blood; it is a part of you, and it is influenced by your thoughts, your perspectives, and your emotions as much as it is affected by what you eat and how many hours you exercise and sleep.

By believing that you are separate from your body, that it's not part of your overall being, you are short-changing yourself and giving up your responsibility and empowerment when it comes to healing. Here is an example. You might have noticed that when you are stressed, you give in to shallow breathing. Yet by mindfully taking deeper and longer breaths, you can alter both your physical and mental state. By changing the rhythm of your breathing, you can restore yourself to equilibrium and grounding. You can defuse stressors by changing the pacing of something you take for granted—your breathing.

In the same way that you don't live in a vacuum, healing doesn't take place in a vacuum. In Soul Healing, I clear your energetic field and negativities that are caught up in your physical body before downloading very high, life-sustaining vibrational frequencies into you.

However, let's say your illness was caused by a lifetime of bottling up your emotions. Your physical symptoms are cleared, you feel more energetic, and you are renewed, but if you resume your tendency to bottle up your emotions, rather than having the courage and confidence to speak your truth, then dis-ease will return in some manner or other in your body.

Soul Healing has its roots in quantum physics, which says we are all part of the Unified Field of Energy that contains all possibilities of realities, and which responds to our thoughts and feelings. Everything is made of energy, and energy vibrates at different frequencies to manifest different states of matter. The higher your cellular vibration, the higher the state of energy, or vice versa, and the more you can empower yourself and live with joy, health, and happiness. Further, every living thing broadcasts a distinct energy pattern, and this pattern carries information. Likewise, when I download a remedy into a client, I am downloading information that puts right the energy pattern of the client.

According to quantum physics, most energy (as much as 90%) is unseen, including the energy or life force in our bodies. For most of you who accept that there is only a 3-dimensional reality, you are purely defined by your physical bodies. In truth, we are multi-dimensional beings made up of our physical, emotional, mental, and spiritual bodies, chakras, and thousands of acupuncture meridians and points, and when any of these selves are out of whack, our entire being is affected.

When you are sick, you are more likely to feel down and pessimistic, but when the life force is flowing strongly in you, it's easier for you to think clearly and feel optimistic. You are a being of many dimensions, and you require a multi-dimensional healing modality. Soul Healing has arrived, and that truth needs to be spoken.

Clearing the Energetics of Relationships

To fully ensure that you stay well and healed, you have to look around at your environment and observe what is negative in your life. For many of you, relationships can be quite a toll on your peace of mind and on your state of health. Relationship conflicts can leave you frazzled and overwhelmed, and leave you insecure and unsure about how to handle other stressful areas of your life.

Whether it is with family or partner or work colleagues, take a close look at whether a certain relationship is beneficial or detrimental to you. When you have identified those that are not constructive, you can make a clean break, or if you can't, then change how you respond to those types of relationships. You may have to forgive those who have hurt you so that you can move forward.

According to the Centre for Addiction and Mental Health (CAMH), psychological distress, which refers to anxiety or depression, has been rising among Ontario students, since 2013, when they started monitoring students in Grades 7 to 12. I had a chance recently to work with a young girl, Alexa O, who suffered depression and anxiety all throughout her teenage years. When she came to me, she had been grappling with her disorders for several years. After one healing, she felt a profound shift. After the second treatment, she described herself to me as feeling very light, positive, and happy.

Then, soon after, she got into a fight with her boyfriend, and she immediately plunged deep into the dumps again. She fell back into victim mode. The conflict and her subsequent retreat into feeling the victim, brought on a big energy leak, and the healing vibrations left her. Before I proceeded with the third healing, I decided to step into a coaching role to have a chat with her, or else the healing sessions would be for naught. We discussed how, by reacting negatively to the conflict with her boyfriend, she was undoing all the good from the previous two sessions, so I encouraged her to be mindful and not to be reactive in her interactions with people.

I underlined the importance of her taking responsibility for her own health, and reacting explosively to any provocation or annoyance with her boyfriend wasn't doing her any good.

She put my advice into practice. It wasn't easy going at first, but she could see how her wellbeing was linked to her emotional state, and she is now able to sustain her happiness. Once in a while, she calls me up for a reboot.

We are a very reactive society in general. We fly off the handle at the smallest slight, and those who are easily angered get so riled up, they shoot at someone who cuts them off on the highways. Road rage is just a symptom of an overly stressed society.

How do we stay grounded, calm, and happy in a high-stress, fast-paced society? These are my suggestions:

- Meditate daily. If you need some encouragement, apps like Calm or Headspace are very easy to use, and help you raise your vibration. Start with short, 5 to 10-minute meditations until you develop a routine.
- Don't take it personally (whatever it may be). Make healthy choices on how to respond to stress and conflict, and establish safe boundaries.
- Live mindfully. Don't rush into the future or even the next minute. Stay in this present moment, and relish the simple joys that are in your life, such as the smell of coffee or tea, or the texture of the porcelain mug in your hand.
- Embrace forgiveness of others, and let go of grudges. If you hold on to a wounding, the wound will never heal, and the pain will never go away. I am not suggesting excusing the harm done, but forgiving, in essence, means letting go of resentment and not harbouring thoughts of hurting the person who injured you.

You can start taking such steps at any age. When my 14-year-old son started meditation, he had a slight headache in the beginning, and that was because the high-level energies were going through him like a force, and his body had to adjust. But he felt energised and simultaneously calm throughout his entire being.

Clearing Your Space

You have probably noticed this. You walk into a place—a meditation retreat, a yoga space, or even a lovely garden—and you feel uplifted or at best at peace. There is something refreshing and soothing about such spaces. Then you step into a conference room in which everyone is unhappy and angry, and the atmosphere feels dense on your skin, as if someone has laid a heavy woollen cape on you, and you just can't breathe.

People leave energy signatures in spaces, and spaces store energy, be they positive or negative. Energy in spaces will fade over time, but if the heightened drama or escalated emotions continue to be replayed in the room, the energy will be anchored to the space. In the same way, when you step into a place of worship, such as a church, a temple or a mosque, a quiet peace infuses the space, and you are bathed in the calming and positive energy, so much so that you want to walk through the space quietly. Few people find it within them to shout and yell in a church—the vibrations just won't support such dense behaviour! A space could have been the scene of a traumatic event, and the energy from that past is now encoded in the energy field of the space.

Negative thoughts, entities, and dark spirits can inhabit a space if they are not cleared. There have been many occasions, when I am about to conduct a healing session or when I am spreading love and light, where something out of the ordinary happens to sabotage my work.

On an occasion, I was helping realign a client at my house. When I discovered hexes and curses on her, the lights explicably went out in my place for three hours. It was as if my house was the point of origin; every neighbour to one side of me was encountering a power outage, whereas the houses on the other side of mine were normally lit. The outage was an indication that I was up against some strong dark forces. Before I could proceed with the session, I had to chat with her to tell her to let go of whatever negativity she was hanging on to, any resentments she had built up against someone, or any anger she was still storing. Negative energies, when fed by continued resentment or despair, will build up, and it was therefore crucial for my client to release and forgive to fully prepare to receive the Divine energies I was about to download into her.

There are ways to clear the energies of a space. Energy can be transferred and transformed, but it cannot be destroyed. It is a form of frequency, like high-pitched sounds that we cannot hear but which are picked up by dogs. Just because we can't see, hear, or touch energy, doesn't mean it doesn't exist. I recommend to occasionally clear your work and home spaces with sage sticks.

You open all windows, light up a stick of sage, and using your hand or a feather, waft the smoke to corners of the room. Smudge dark places like the back of a closet and under the bed for a thorough space cleansing. Native Americans and Canadian First Nations, as well as indigenous tribes in many parts of the world, use smudging because they believe the life force of the smoke absorbs dense, heavy energies. From a scientific perspective, medicinal smoke has been shown to reduce bacteria in the air by an astounding 94%, and keeps the space purer and disinfected for 24 hours.[5]

I recommend to my clients to carry out such steps if I feel they need additional support outside of healing. Within the realm of healing, however, it is not necessary for me to do so. I enter into such a high vibrational state that it surpasses any form of evil or negativity, and in this state, I align the client's body to the energy fields of the Universe and Mother Earth. When energetically cleared and aligned, it is the client's own soul and body that does the healing.

Clearing Mind Programmes

When a client proves resistant to healing, we have to examine what mind programmes he or she has that are tampering with the healing process. Is the person feeling unworthy? Does he hold the belief that his illness is the result of him not being good enough? Does she subscribe to the thought that because other women in her family have suffered this illness, she is not spared from it either?

---

[5] Medicinal smoke reduces airborne bacteria,
https://www.ncbi.nlm.nih.gov/pubmed/17913417

It is in such cases necessary to revisit those areas of a person's life that is impeding the realignment to full health. One way I can help alter the client's perspective is to get them still, move them out of thinking only with logic and rationale, and shift them to their heart, for them to get in touch with their feelings. The heart has intuitive intelligence, and it processes far more cognitive information than the brain does. Through the information highway, which is the vagus nerve, the heart sends more signals to the brain than the brain to the heart. In essence, trust that the heart knows exactly what it is doing.

Empowering Yourself to Heal

I cannot stress enough that your health is your own responsibility. Clients like Alexa O, who have trouble mastering their emotions, are tempted to pin the responsibility for their health on me. No, that is not my job; my job is to get you started on your healing journey by restoring your energetic patterning to its right state.

But as mentioned before, energy can be transformed, and if you continue to put up with dysfunctional relationships, toxic work environments, or unhealthy living spaces, your healing will be short-circuited. In addition to coming to me for a Soul Healing, it's up to you to examine what areas of your life need to be addressed or put right. I will often provide coaching tips when I see that the client will benefit from my suggestions. In the end, my role is to empower your own healing.

Soul Healing is appearing at a time when millions of people are not getting adequate medical care because of spiralling medical and pharmaceutical costs, long lines at emergency, and understaffed and underequipped hospitals. There are horror stories of people who have unfortunately been stuck with huge emergency bills that are not covered by their insurance. Insurance companies are getting increasingly fussy about offering sufficient coverage, and in some cases, existing illnesses fall outside of coverage. Further, insurance coverage stops once you reach a certain age; it's unfortunate that people are being financially punished for living longer. People are demanding solutions so they can live more productive and longer lives.

Let me ask you this. Which do you prefer? A lifetime of visiting hospitals, increasing number of prescriptions and escalating pharmaceutical costs, confined to a walker or wheelchair, or a simple, 4-step Soul Healing?

7
Words Have Power

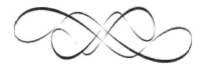

"Words have energy and power with the ability to help, to heal, to hinder, to hurt, to harm, to humiliate, and to humble."
– Yehuda Berg

Words can heal and words can kill. Words pack power; they carry energy, and they are vessels for the raw materials of manifestation. That's why it's necessary to choose your words with care, and to speak only words of power, inspiration, love, compassion, and truth.

Words are powerful containers of energy, and they can be used to rouse a mob to destruction or to inspire a crowd with greatness. What you say matters to the people around you because, as author Gary Chapman says in his book, *Love as a Way of Life*, words can be either "bullets or seeds." What are you sowing in the minds of another when you speak? Are you sowing seeds of trust, of honesty and of hope, or are you smashing their dreams and desires with bullets?

We can choose to use this force constructively with words of encouragement, or destructively with words of despair.

There is a reason for the phrase "cutting words," because someone who lashes out angrily will use words that cut into your energetic field, and if you are highly sensitive, you might even feel it as a slap on your body. Yet when someone speaks encouraging words that stir and motivate, you would feel an infusion of energy that makes you feel as if you are ready to conquer the world.

So, why aren't people more careful with the words they speak? Because they don't understand that words are forces of energy.

Let's try this simple experiment. I reproduced below, two famous poems, and it will be interesting for you to note which emotions surface and for which piece.

Here is a poem by the Greek poet, Homer, written more than two thousand years ago.

"I will sing of well-founded Earth, mother of all, eldest of all beings.
She feeds all creatures that are in the world, all that go upon the
goodly land, and all that are in the paths of the seas,
and all that fly:
all these are fed of her store."

How did those lines make you feel? Each time I read them, they fill me with gratitude that we have this beautiful blue planet Earth to call home, to feed, and to take care of us.

Here is an extract from another poem, from a different era and circumstances.

Take up our quarrel with the foe:
To you from failing hands we throw
The torch; be yours to hold it high.

If ye break faith with us who die
We shall not sleep, though poppies grow
In Flanders fields.

This poem, In Flanders Field, by Canadian war poet, John McCrae, imbues me with great sadness that so many young lives were lost, and so many dreams are extinguished when men go to war. How did you feel? Were the emotions that were aroused different from the ones that surfaced when you read Homer's poem?

It's not just the words you say that are important. It's also the words you think that are affecting you. What you say and think are affecting you internally. The words you utter and the words you mull over, or the ones that are playing over and over again in your mind, are impacting your cells—all 75 trillion of them— that listen in to your every word. As part of the new biology advocated by authorities such as Dr. Bruce Lipton, your cells are being shaped by the environment, and whatever you broadcast to them will affect the cell programming. Your cell's genes contain myriad possibilities, but the potential that does manifest depends on the information you are sending to it.

If you tell yourself every day that you are aging, your cells will hear you, and it won't be too long before more gray appears in your hair, more wrinkles appear on your face, and you don't feel as strong as you did when you were in your 30s. If you say that you are sad in conversation, and think sad thoughts, your cells hear you, and they say, "She wants to be sad; let's give her more of it," and your body slows down, you become less mobile and sociable, and you become even more reclusive.

You are not just a function of your genes. It's outmoded thinking to believe that your genes make your body and your life. Your cells absorb the information and vibes you are sending to it, and what is manifested depends on what you say to them. You literally speak things into being.

Your body is a miracle that was designed to heal itself. It has an innate intelligence that powers you and your life without your being aware of it. Did you know that a single neuron, the bit that transmits information from the brain to all parts of your body, can handle as many as 833 impulses or signals every second, and that just your brain alone has 86 billion neurons? Are you aware that your liver performs 500 different functions without you consciously telling it to do so? And this complex, wondrous body started out from just two cells, one from each parent?

That's why you hear stories of miraculous healing, where patients heal by inwardly engaging with their bodies. Let's look at this, one step at a time. Stress is now so endemic that it is now believed to be the silent killer, but how does stress manifest in you? It is brought on by how you perceive and react to a situation, and those emotions trigger a release of biochemicals that help a fight or flight reaction. But when you are in chronic stress, the biochemicals that are unrelentingly released, chip away at your immune system, weakening your resistance to infections and diseases.

The stress hormones, such as adrenalin and cortisol, which are released to cope with stress, are meant only to handle short-term situations. However, when your stress response goes wild and is switched on all the time, your overexposure to these hormones throws your digestive tract out of whack, weakens your heart, and makes you vulnerable to strokes and other heart diseases, as well as anxiety and depression.

If your body reacts negatively to negative emotions, surely it stands to reason that it will react positively to positive emotions, which in turn are brought on by happy situations and positive words. I encourage you to use positive affirmations to disrupt the negative thoughts that feed your anxiety and emotional imbalance.

Speak kindly to yourself, and life will seem better. Speak kindly to others, and you will find community. I am not saying to suppress the truth or lie, but even in situations of conflict, you can use positive words to defuse the tension and to invite mindfulness on the part of each of the participants.

We live in interesting times, where there is increasing understanding and recognition that words have the power to shape our reality. You can see the impact in our social cultures. Words such as *disabled* are being replaced by terms such as *differently-abled,* because language is now acknowledging that people are not defined by their handicaps. In health care, the emergence of person-centred care is redefining how patients are described. A person with dementia is no longer a demented patient but a patient suffering from dementia.

Words Can Programme Water, They Can Programme Your Body

You must have heard about experiments by Japanese scientist, Dr. Masaru Emoto, who found that water molecules reacted to the words that were thrown at them. He put water in several different glasses and wrote different words on each of the containers. Water molecules from those glasses labelled with positive words like *love, peace, harmony,* and *thank you,* produced beautifully formed, colourful, and complex snowflake-like crystals, which were revealed using high-speed photography. In sharp contrast, water taken from the containers labelled with negative words, such as *hate, you disgust me,* and *I hate you,* showed distorted, asymmetrical, and colourless patterns.

His research, which spanned twenty years, also reveals that polluted and toxic water can be purified and restored when exposed to prayer and harmonious intentions. In his book, *Messages from Water,* he showed two slides of water molecules from the Fujiwara Dam in Japan. In its polluted state, the crystals were shapeless and ugly. He then took pictures of water from the same dam after the chief priest of Jyuhouin Temple, the Reverend Kato Hoki, prayed for an hour over the dam. The water crystal was ornate, symmetrical, and beautiful in shape and pattern.

Have you noticed how great you feel when you stand by a pristine waterfall in the jungle, or when you swim in its pool? What about when you drink clear, spring water from the source? You can feel its sweetness, and you likely feel very refreshed. In both these cases, the water crystals are harmonious and beautiful in shape, and they carry that vibration into you.

Here is the revelation, which has very important implications for your healing and for world harmony. Your bodies are nearly 80% water, so you too are definitely affected by the words that are flung at you, the words that you think, and the words that you use. The water in your cells reacts to the frequency of the words around you, and the molecules form shapes in resonance with those frequencies.

You may think that this is unbelievable, but human consciousness has a direct impact on water. Your consciousness (in your words, your thoughts, and emotions) imprints and transforms water. Ask yourself these questions in the light of this information. Are you polluting your body and your health with your words and the words of the company you keep, or are you blessing your body with the frequencies of beautiful and uplifting words?

That is the reason why, when I conduct a Soul Healing, I place a cup of water next to the client. As the client receives the high-level vibrations that I download, so will the cup of water, which he or she drinks after the session is over. That was how I healed from a debilitating ankle injury, and it was that very same event that compelled me to learn more about Soul Healing. I do the same when I conduct a long-distance healing or when I conduct Soul Healing through a podcast. I recommend to all my clients to have a glass of water within easy reach, because the water will be imprinted with the purity and goodness of the Universal Force, and will carry the healing frequencies into my patients' bodies.

Mantras for Healing

You may have heard of mantras but never really understood what they are for and how they work. Since words and thoughts are shown to have an impact on your life and health, why not choose the ones that are elevating, uplifting, and expansive?

Mantra is a Sanskrit word derived from two root words: *manas* meaning the linear thinking mind, and *tra*, which means to cross over. Mantras are sacred sounds and words used in old, spiritual traditions, and practised by early Hinduism and Buddhism practitioners.

Mantras are thought of as a way of using sound to cut through the mental chaos in your mind, change your state of mind, and to connect "directly and immediately to deep states of energy and consciousness."[6]

The reality that you now live in is created by the words you have spoken and the thoughts you previously voiced silently in your mind, so why not create a more positive and life-enhancing life from now onwards? You don't have to be practising a specific religion to use mantras, because they cut

---

[6] Russill Paul, The Yoga of Sound: Tapping the Hidden Power of Music and Chant.

across religious lines, and thrive on the energy of sound to connect to the Universe.

The mantras have vibrations unique to themselves, and they accelerate inner awakening, retraining of the subconscious mind, laying the tracks for new thought patterns and paving the way to manifest good in your life. When you repeat or sing the mantras, your intention is as important as the words. Mantras are just a string of words, but you turbo-boost them by adding intention and belief to them. That's when the magic starts to work—because by immersing your whole body into the feeling of the words, you amp up the effectiveness of the sayings, and strengthen your connection to a higher power.

Be patient; give yourself time to reap the benefits of the mantras. You are undoing and untangling years of unwelcomed, self-deprecating inner negativity, so it only stands to reason that you should give yourself some time for the positivity and healing forces to flow into your life.

Don't underestimate the hidden power of words. When you are down on yourself, the words that come to mind are negative, and you are permitting the power of words to work against you. Consciously choose the words that uplift, elevate, and transform, and choose with care the emotional force with which you express them. Your ability to heal and thrive depends on the words you seek out, the words you express, and the words you receive.

Here are a few of the mantras that I recommend to my clients for their daily affirmation practice:

- I deserve a good life.
- I am open.
- I love and respect myself.
- I forgive myself.
- I have inner peace and have unconditional love for myself and others.
- I trust in the Universe. The Universe always has my back.
- I am worthy of good things.
- I have the power to heal myself anytime I want, and I can access the universal energy field and don't need anyone to heal me.
- I am abundant in all ways... health, wealth, and happiness.
- I am enough.
- I will stay true to who I am.
- I deserve the love I am given.
- I choose me.
- Any obstacle, whether it be a person or situation, is designed for me to expand my soul.
- How can it get any better than this?
- What else is possible?

It is important not to let this become a chore. Infuse your mantras with belief, feeling, and intention. Mantras are meant to be uplifting and joyful, and if it helps, you can repeat them softly, recite them out loud, or write them out on sticky notes that you can look at often. Wear clothes that have positive phrases or mantras on them. Use the power of repetition to consciously shift the way you live your life.

Be aware of throw-away words, such as "I dislike my body," or "I hate myself." How many times a day do you do that to yourself?

Words can give you wings, so dedicate some time to better use them every day. Start the day with a healthy diet of awesome mantras, and you'll be surprised how pleasant the day will turn out to be. Of course, you will have bad days. But rather than dwelling on bad moments and making them worse by overthinking about it, take note of the obstacles, make appropriate adjustments, and get back on track with your mantras.

Finally, I would like to mention that the words you receive and which are flung your way will have an impact on you. There are some people who are simply toxic and who take delight in using their words to cut, to bully, and to manipulate others. Your choices with these people are simple. Move on without them, speak up, and defend your boundaries; don't take it personally, and give yourself self-care by making time for yourself, free of toxic people and toxic words.

Leverage the power of words to work for you, not against you.

8
Forgive Easily,
Be Grateful Constantly

"In the vibration of appreciation, all things come to you.
You don't have to make anything happen."
– Esther Hicks

Forgiveness is a deliberate conscious act of love. It is a decision made to stop holding on to anger, resentment, or even hate for someone or something, or even for the self. Forgiveness is an act of self-love because, by not letting go, the anger grows and grows, and over the years takes up so much space in your energy field, there is no room to let in anything else.

But it is so common for us to hold on to past resentments. By doing so, we replay over and over again in our heads the event that caused us to be first angry, and we relive each and every feeling of hurt, despair, and disappointment that we felt then. And we feel it so strongly and so vividly as if the precipitating event is happening right here and now. In the meantime, this increasingly growing ball of energy (or several balls of them if you are nursing several grudges) is playing havoc with your outlook on life, your health, and your emotional well-being.

Nursing a resentment means you are always looking backwards into the past, because that is what's claiming your attention right now, and in the process, you forgo and lose the wonder and power of living in the moment, and you are shut off from any positive energies and opportunities that are making their way to you.

So why do you hold on to grudges? Is it because you feel that you are getting control of the situation by harbouring the resentment? Maybe it would help if you better understood what forgiveness really involves:

- Forgiveness doesn't mean reconciliation.
- Forgiveness doesn't mean you let the other person get away scot-free.
- Forgiveness doesn't mean you have to put up with the same negative behavior or abuse from the other person.
- Forgiveness means giving yourself permission to stop playing the victim.
- Forgiveness means loving yourself enough to let go of something that lowers your energy and vibration.
- Forgiveness is a choice and a decision to live to your highest potential, not to be held back by past roadblocks and obstacles.

Not Forgiving Messes Up Your Health

As a Soul Healer, I have seen how resentments and grudges lodge themselves in a person's body. They manifest in disorders like anxiety, depression, back pain, and chronic illnesses.

In Chapter 6, *Steps of Healing*, I brought up the case of Alexa O, who had suffered depression throughout her teen years.

Teenage depression is a growing problem, and one in 8 adolescents get depressed and suffer multiple associated problems, including memory loss, anxiety, difficulty making decisions, and excessive irresponsibility. Whatever were the causes in Alexa's case, her healing became sustained when she forgave the toxic relationships in her life, and made peace with the people in whatever way she could.

Even though she felt a distinct and positive change after the first and second Soul Healing sessions with me, memories of her unhappy relationships still clung to her like barnacles. When she finally understood that forgiveness was the last piece of the puzzle that she needed in order to sustain the high vibrations from Soul Healing, that was the moment she fully healed.

From Forgiveness to Gratitude

On the flip side of forgiveness is gratitude. When your energy field is no longer warped and twisted by resentments, you are able to see what is good in your life and express gratitude for it. What does gratitude mean to you? Gratitude focuses your attention on the positives in your life and being thankful for what you have. Not just for the big things like a new house or a job promotion, but for the simplest joys, like waking up to the smell of coffee in the morning, or being able to have a hot shower before setting out for the day.

Gratitude takes you away from toxic emotions like envy and resentment, because when you are so filled with joy for the blessings you have, there is simply no room for negativity. Studies[7] show that gratitude rewires the brain and enhances your mental health, and I should add, it transforms the rest of your being. You are healthier, you handle stress better, you have clarity when challenges arise, and you come up with solutions.

All in all, gratitude puts you in a very good place. This is simply because gratitude is an affirmation of goodness—an acknowledgement of the good things you have received, the supportive relationships you have in your life, and a deep appreciation for who you are.

Resentment increases resistance in your life, so that even if good things are flowing towards you, they have a hard time getting to you as they have to find ways around the energetic blocks, just like water winds its way around rocks and pebbles in a stream. Gratitude, on the other hand, speeds up manifestation, because as you well know, you attract what you beam out energetically.

When you exude delight, joy, and gratitude, the Universe sends back to you even more to be delighted about and joyful and grateful for. The stronger the feelings, the more potent and faster is the manifestation. The more you feel your desires as if they are already manifested in your body, the speedier will the Universe answer you. Try it. In the next moment, describe five things that you are grateful for. Find

---

[7] https://greatergood.berkeley.edu/article/item/how_gratitude_changes_you _and_your_brain

five people that you are thankful to have in your life. At the end of every day before you go to sleep, say thanks for a day of accomplishment, or downtime (whatever the case may be), and when you wake, before you get out of bed, say that you are grateful for a brand new day in which to create and to do good.

Create Your Desires

Gratitude doesn't mean that you stop dreaming and visioning for new things to come into your life. On the contrary, when you are grateful, the Universe hears you and will send you more to be grateful for, in surprising and unexpected ways. When you are grateful, you are plugged into the Creative Source. Doors will open, miracles will come, and life lines up in your favour. And in turn, you become a positive and healing influence on the world.

Be grateful for what you now have, and keep on desiring. The Universe wants you to create your desires because that is how you are designed to live—to create in partnership with the Universe.

That's how I started on this life-changing trajectory. I joined a podcast by Ed Strachar, received a long-distance healing, and although his week-long course in Phoenix seemed too expensive, my desire was so pure and undiluted that the Universe opened up doors to me. Without me asking, my family came around to support me financially.

And here I am, offering the world a revolutionary modality, Soul Healing, and empowering people to take better care of themselves. I have come a long way from pharmacy school, 30 years ago. I still love my pharmacy practice, but I have always desired to offer both conventional medicine and alternative and natural therapies. Now I am at the bleeding edge of vibrational medicine.

The Universe is expanding every second, and you have to grow in your potential along with it. You make different choices when you are in a state of gratitude than when you are caught up in anxiety, frustration, or anger. When you are humming along on the gratitude frequency, you will find that the Universe is not only a co-creator, it's your biggest ally.

Forgive easily; be grateful constantly.

9
Love Rules

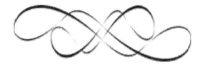

*"Eventually you will come to understand that love heals
everything, and love is all there is."*
– Gary Zukav

Love is the most powerful force in the Universe. That I am
sure you will agree with me. There are all sorts of reasons as
to why love is so powerful and potent, but there is so much
truth in the saying "love conquers all." It most certainly does.
Now, if we want to throw some science and spiritual wisdom
into the mix, one reason behind its power is that love has a
frequency, 528 Hz, which resonates at the heart of the matrix
of creation, and it connects us to the Creative Source. It is
also the most powerful healing force on the planet, because
its frequency and vibrations are stronger than every other
emotion that we feel.

Love heals because its frequency helps you to flow in perfect
rhythm and inner harmony, and when you are aligned with
Universal Flow, you are healthy. It's quite simple. In the
words of spiritual teacher, psychiatrist, and author, Dr.
David Hawkins, "A loving thought then heals, and a
negative thought creates illness. Choosing to become a
loving person results in the release of endorphins by the
brain, which has a profound effect on the body's health and
happiness."

You don't need a lot of scientific literature to feel the difference between love and fear. When you are in love, the world feels right, everything sparkles, possibilities abound and your cells are humming along. When you feel fear, you feel a disturbance in your gut, and if the feeling persists, your body shuts down to protect you from outside negative influences. What happens when you live in a constant state of fear—be it linked to stress, anxiety, a lack of support, or depression—is that over the long term, fear shuts down the body. It compromises the immune system and bolts down all the functions related to the growth and maintenance of the body. The end result? Disease.

When your body feels love, everything runs smoothly; your body is maintained, and the immune system operates at peak level. So is falling in love then the key to healing?

Love is multi-faced. There is romantic love, parental love, love of family, love of a country, love of pets, love of arts, and the list goes on. I would venture that when it comes to healing, self-love is one of the most important expressions of love for anyone.

A lot goes wrong in the world when a person doesn't feel deserving of love. Those who don't feel self-love are prone to any number of ills, including addiction. That's because they use addictive substances to drown out feelings of unworthiness, to quiet the self-judgment that they are less than others, and to disaffirm their entrenched belief that their life is one of struggle.

In order for any healing to work, including Soul Healing, you need to feel that you deserve optimal health, and you need to be open to receiving love. When you don't love yourself, you don't take care of yourself. When you don't exercise self-care, you suffer. However, when you don't take care of yourself, you are not the only person who suffers. Others suffer with you too, and these include the people in your life who are depending on you. These people are expecting you to be healthy across the board—spiritually, physically, mentally, and emotionally.

Soul Healing works on highest-level vibrations and frequencies, and if you are not capable of welcoming love into your life, you just won't receive the healing frequency of love. Even when I successfully download the healing energies into you, your inability to accept the healing is tantamount to an energy leak. And as previously discussed, energy leaks cause the high-level frequencies to drain from your field, cancelling any of the positive results of Soul Healing. And you are back to where you first started, with your health problems.

But when you let love into your life, you heal all wounds, whether they are physical, mental, or emotional, or past or present.

I have a pretty good relationship with my first ex-husband, Antonio, the father of my first son, Andreas. He has always had my back. Once, he travelled from Florida to see his son, and he told me that he was suffering migraines all day long, till one in the morning. He works in the restaurant industry in Florida, and when I tested him, I found that he had a lot of demons in his field. So I cleared his energy field of all forms of negativity, and the next morning, he said that he felt a slight dizziness but was no longer suffering migraines.

However, he had a few glasses of wine, and the alcohol created a huge energy leak, so he found himself susceptible to migraines again. I carried out a second treatment on him and strongly advised him to stop drinking. I explained to him that even cutting down to one to two glasses a day would lower the energy of the body, and make it vulnerable to negative forces again.

He took my recommendation to heart and, as a result of staying off alcohol, he has lost 10 lbs out of a necessary weight loss of 30 lbs, and feels so much better. Although we are no longer together, love overcomes any past wounding, and I will always take care of him and the people around him.

When Antonio was in town, I conducted a Soul Healing on a group, which included past and present family members: Antonio; my son, Andreas; and his then girlfriend, who suffered bad allergic reactions from eating any rice, wheat, or dairy. Since the Soul Healing, her food allergies have been mitigated, and she is also more circumspect about her diet.

However, there is an underside to love, which exposes itself when love becomes over-protective or over-controlling.

Not too long ago, a woman in her 40s walked into my pharmacy. I am certified in Ontario to be a specialist in providing information on marijuana—*cannabidiol* (CBD) and *tetrahydrocannabinol* (THC), the psychoactive element of marijuana. A woman came in to have a discovery session with me. However, while we were chatting, she checked out my Facebook profile, read that I offered Soul Healing, and asked if I would conduct a healing on her on the spot.

It wasn't something I like to do ordinarily, but I thought to give her a brief introduction to the energies of Soul Healing. I cleared her field and was just downloading the high-level energies into her. But as a practicing yogi, she was far more open, sensitive, and attuned to energy healing than the ordinary person. Before too long, she was quivering from the high-energy downloads. I stopped because I felt that she had enough. For many of my clients, they will feel reenergised gradually throughout the course of the session, but she got it right away.

When I ended the download, she continued our conversation and said that she had gained a lot of clarity about the personal challenges she was going through. She expressed great concern about her teenage daughter, whom she felt was suffering through depression, and as a loving mother, wanted me to heal the daughter. But she felt she needed to try out Soul Healing for herself first.

I, however, advised her differently. The umbilical cord that tied a mother to a baby during pregnancy still exists energetically, and the more the mother worried about her daughter, the more likely she was worsening her daughter's depression. She may not express anything of her concern outright to her daughter, but even if she puts on a happy face, her internal distress will be felt through the energetic umbilical cord. The more energy she invested into worrying about her kid, the more she was driving her kid away.

I told her that in order to heal her daughter, she had to first heal herself. Currently, each time she thought of her daughter, her thoughts were accompanied by feelings of imbalance, depression, and lack, further aggravating the energy of deficit that both of them felt around the teenager's emotional state. Where the mother needed healing was to not invest in those negative energies any further, but to change her internal mind-set to only focus on seeing her daughter as a healed, happy, and healthy teenager.

This was the same advice I gave Quinn's mother. Quinn was the young boy whose mother called me up at midnight when he was suffering from gastroenteritis (see Chapter 5). His mom tended to be a worrier, and I advised her that everyone in her family would be better off if I did a Soul Healing on her to erase any past traumas that might have led to her needing to excessively protect her son. If she continued on her current path, the negative consequence would be that her over-anxiety would rub off on her children, who might grow up without a robust sense of self-esteem or self-resiliency. Soul Healing would remove any of her ingrained patterns of behaviour, and help her visualize and create a new path to bring forth what she really wanted of her family and herself.

Side-Effects of Soul Healing

It's an interesting observation that many of my clients who have benefitted from Soul Healing find a need to clean up other areas of their lives. It's almost as if the remaining shadows of their lives need to come up for air, as if they are pulled up from the dark recesses by the Divine Light that is downloaded into them. On another occasion, a new client confessed that she was having problems with her husband, and she felt that her marriage was on the rocks. They were, however, planning to go away for an extended weekend to see if they could work things out, and she asked for some advice on what to do.

It was really quite simple, I told her, and set her a little task. During their weekend away, she had only to think about and focus on what she liked or enjoyed about her husband. If she could only find three things she enjoyed about him, and five things she didn't, for the course of the weekend, she had to only focus on those three positive things and shelve the others aside. By doing so, she would raise her vibration, and the rest would follow suit and fix themselves.

It is not an easy thing to abandon years of patterning, and switch gears like that. Changing your mind-set requires conscious and deliberate effort, just like you would need time to build a muscle in the gym.

I also reminded her that it wasn't her husband's job to make her happy, nor was it his responsibility to have to respond to her neediness. Happiness was her own responsibility, and rather than seeing her husband as the solution to her problems, she needed to view him as a co-creator with whom she could build a strong marriage and relationship.

The greatest of marriages won't fix you if you are simply not happy with yourself. That's where self-love comes in. You can only fully love another if you are happy with yourself, or else you'll project your unhappiness onto your partner and expect him or her to fix you. And it's important to always focus on what's good and working about the relationship, rather than to highlight the bad, because then the bad will overwhelm the good. It can be the other way around.

This particular client came back to me after the weekend and requested another healing session. I like to space my sessions at least a week apart, and advised her to wait. Healing sometimes takes time to manifest; it also depends on how much effort my clients put into the post-session exercises I give them to properly seal in the elevated vibrations.

Making Self-Love a Priority for True Healing

Soul Healing is revolutionary, but we are in an age of accelerated consciousness, which demands a new way of being now and in the future. The time for Soul Healing has come; its results are powerful, profound, and life changing. I am a healer, and I see that my mission is to empower others to heal themselves— emotionally, physically, and spiritually—by offering a new, powerful method of healing for a new, powerful way of life.

Throughout this book and on my website, www.drugsto distanthealing.com, I have given you a few tools to get you started on healing your life. Here are a few more because, as this is the final chapter and it's about love, I consider it essential that you start first with self-love. Life becomes easier when you choose to love and honour yourself your way.

- **Forgive yourself** – You can choose to be shackled to past resentments or feelings of guilt related to past incidents, and they will always be baggage that you carry throughout your life. Or you can forgive yourself, accept who you are, and move forward confidently, without the extra weight of past guilt. What's good about self-forgiveness is that when you are yourself free from blame, you are better able to accept others as they are.

- **Select the company you hang out with** – Don't give in to those who gain by pulling you down to their level. That's just them projecting their own lack of self-worth on you. But in order to love yourself, you need to put some distance between you and those who put you down. Seek out only those who inspire and motivate you.

- **Make the changes you need now** – Take small steps, but take them immediately. It's the rest of your life we are talking about. Your life, till now, is the result of the steps you've taken in the past, and if you want it to be any different in the future, you have to act and think differently. Change happens first at the level of thought and then action. Don't wait. It's your happiness at stake.

Find me at **www.drugstodistanthealing.com.** Let's chat about healing yourself with Soul Healing. You can get a bonus meditation to help you get started on this new, exciting journey ahead of you, to remake yourself as you wish to be.

Appendix
Alternative and Natural Remedies

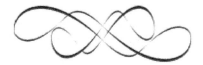

"Nurturing yourself is not selfish—it's essential to your survival and your well-being."
– Renee Peterson Trudeau

Healing doesn't have to be difficult. In fact, healing should be and can be very simple. Right now, with alternative remedies gaining mainstream respectability, with many medical insurance companies willing to cover some alternative therapies, we have many choices to pick from. Natural remedies may seem new and revolutionary to many people, but in truth, many of them have been practiced for thousands of years.

Alternative remedies focus on the holistic approach, i.e. treating the entire person—the mind, body, and spirit. We are arriving at a new understanding of how to handle our health. It is a profound transformation; there is a fundamental shift in how we view taking care of ourselves, and it is up to us to acquaint ourselves with the various alternative remedies to better understand our choices.

I spent 10 years after starting my pharmacy, exploring a wide range of alternative healing modalities. In this chapter, I seek to touch briefly on various modalities in alternative and natural remedies. Each of these eight categories deserve their own book, but my purpose here is to offer an introduction to those for whom alternative remedies are as yet unknown or unfamiliar. They are:

- Herbs and spices
- Homeopathy
- Flower essences
- Acupuncture
- Bio-intolerance elimination
- Quantum machines
- Colour therapy and gemstones
- Meditation

Herbs and Spices

Herbalism or healing with plants has deep roots in the past but is now being viewed with new understanding. Herbs are those plants that do not have any woody fibres but whose stems are soft and pliable. Herbs can be derived from the whole plant, the leaves, flowers, or even just the roots. Such plants can be used on any condition that is medically treatable, and what is interesting is that herbs deliver more antioxidants than fruits or vegetables, based on weight. Herbs and spices have many phytochemicals, many of which act as powerful antioxidants that help strengthen our innate healing abilities. The substance in herbs that has the most potent antioxidant activity, and therefore is excellent for anti-inflammation, is a phenol component called rosmarinic acid. This particular phenol is present in many plants in the Lamiaceae family, including rosemary, sage, oregano, and lemon balm.

The list below is not meant to be an exhaustive list of healing herbs and spices. It is meant instead to give you a sense of how diverse healing herbs can be, and is a good place for you to get started. Instead of reaching for your salt shaker at dinner time, grab some herbs to sprinkle on your food to boost flavours and add healthy anti-inflammatory properties. Alternatively, you can steep a handful of herbs for a relaxing and healthy cup of tea.

Echinacea
Part of the daisy family, Echinacea is used as an immune system strengthener and to prevent colds and flus.

St. John's Wort
A herb with yellow flowers, St. John's Wort grows in the wild and has been traditionally used for treating mental illnesses, and is popularly used to help patients suffering from mild to moderate depression.

Milk Thistle
More powerful as an antioxidant than Vitamin C, it contains silymarin, which is a substance that helps to regenerate already damaged liver tissue, and offers protection from alcohol, drugs, pollution, and free radical damage.

Oregano
Oregano has between three and twenty times more antioxidant strength than 33 other herbs studied by researchers in the US Department of Agriculture. Here are some interesting numbers. One gram of oregano gets you

four times more antioxidant activity than a gram of blueberries, and 42 times more than in one gram of apple.

Rosemary
Much of the anti-inflammation properties in rosemary comes from rosmarinic acid, as well as compounds shared with sage. These compounds heal by boosting the work of any enzyme that removes superoxide, a powerful free radical that is thought to cause chronic inflammation.

Turmeric
A spice that packs a mighty punch, the component in turmeric that is the anti-inflammation warrior is curcumin. Curcumin gives turmeric its golden yellow colour, and it is shown to restrict tumour cell growth in different types of cancer and improves insulin resistance in patients with abnormal metabolic functions.

Homeopathy

Worldwide, there are 200 million users of homeopathics, and homeopathy is included in the national health systems of countries like Brazil, Chile, India, Mexico, Pakistan and Switzerland, according to the Homeopathy Research Institute.[8]

---

[8] Homeopathy Research Institute, https://www.hri-research.org/resources/essentialevidence/use-of-homeopathy-across-the-world/

Homeopathy takes that the body knows exactly what it is doing. It is always seeking balance and harmony, like a boat righting itself on the ocean. Symptoms, such as fever, coughing, or mucus production, are signs that the body is taking steps to overcome a problem. The homeopath believes that the patient is cured by finding a remedy that produces the very same symptoms the patient is recovering. Remedies undergo various rounds of dilution and shaking so that they are non-invasive, non-toxic, and without side effects.

Homeopathy is holistic in nature, and the homeopath considers the patient's mind, body, and spirit, the whole person, in making recommendations. Homeopathics are made from natural substances: vegetable, minerals, and animal.

Flower Essences

It was Welsh physician, Dr. Edward Bach, who discovered the 38 flowers and trees that relieved emotional difficulties, because he believed that true healing treated the true cause of disease, which are emotional and mental in origin. Flower essences work to stabilize emotional and mental stress, and restore balance so that the underlying causes of illness can be treated more easily.

The benefits of flower essences are subtle in nature, and unlike the quick fix of symptoms that come with a pill, the benefits may take a while to show through. But one day, the patient being treated with flower essences may find that he or she is not as stressed out or as anxious, and is not resorting to stress eating, thereby lowering the risk of future heart attacks or diabetes.

Flowers are nature's tools for body wellness and healing. Practitioners of flower essences work on using essences to heal the emotions, which will in turn allow the body to heal itself.

One of the most popular remedies is Rescue Remedy.

Colour Therapy and Gemstones

Most of us brighten up when we dress in colourful clothes. Yellow is energising, red can come across as empowering and fiery, and white as serene and calming. Colour therapy, or chromotherapy, uses the light and colours that are visible to the eye to affect a person's mood and physical or mental health.

The premise behind colour therapy is that the colours contain their own unique frequencies and vibrations, and as these colours enter the body, they activate certain hormones that trigger chemical reactions within the body, which balance emotions and enable the body to heal. Different coloured lights have different wavelengths; as such, some colours are better for skin surface ailments, while others penetrate more deeply into the body.

Gemstone therapy works on the premise that crystals and other stones act as conduits for healing. By placing gemstones on the body, they dissipate blockages and cause negative energies to flow out, and positive, nurturing energy to flow in. The stones are placed on specific points on the body, either on chakras based on the Hindu system of energy systems, or on qi meridians that are intrinsic to Chinese acupuncture.

Acupuncture

Practised for thousands of years, acupuncture is becoming a mainstream therapy. In acupuncture, needles are inserted at specific points in the body to remove blockages and stimulate energy flow, and is used for a wide variety of ailments, from health maintenance to pain-relief to chronic conditions.

Acupuncturists believe inner "qi" travels along energy highways or meridians within the body. There are 12 major meridians (some acupuncturist texts identify 14), which are linked to specific organs and 361 acupuncture points.

Although it is a network of interconnected points like the body's blood circulation system, the meridians are not visible to us. Nonetheless, researchers using systems such as CT scans and MRIs have detected certain features on those sites identified as acupuncture points. These sites have a higher density of clusters of micro-vessels, which are the smallest blood vessels in the body that distribute blood within tissues.

Quantum Machines

We live in the age of energy, and the findings of quantum physics have led to the emergence of quantum machines. These combine state-of-the-art technology with our understanding of quantum physics, and offers healing without invasive surgery or drugs that may cause side effects. Quantum medicine practitioners believe that every cell vibrates to a unique frequency, each of which can be thrown off by internal factors such as stress or poor nutrition, or external factors like environmental pollution.

These machines are designed to accurately detect changes in the quantum frequencies of the cells, and to infuse the body with quantum waves to revert the body's frequencies to their optimal states. The machine conducts a scan, looks at every cell, tissue, and organ of the body, and compares it to a library of optimal frequencies to determine what the stressors are in the body. Stressors can be anything, from energy blockages to allergies, toxins, viruses, or even negative feelings.

I use the Core Inergetix machine to maintain the positive benefits of Soul Healing, when a client requires the additional support.

Bio-Intolerance Elimination

Allergies have been rising at a noticeable rate and, nowadays, one out of every three persons in North America is affected by allergies or some kind of intolerance.

Increasingly, people are turning to alternative remedies since over-the-counter drugs like antihistamines only address the symptoms, not the underlying cause of the problem.

Founded in 1998, BIE shares the belief, as in acupuncture, that blockages can occur in the energetic pathways of the body. These blockages stop the brain and nervous system from receiving the right information about foods or environmental substances, and create a state of confusion. An allergy develops.

BIE uses biofeedback or muscle response testing to establish whether a particular substance (food, pollen, or heavy metals allergens) has resonance or dissonance with the body. Once a specific allergen is identified, the next step is to reprogram cells by transmitting a low electronic frequency onto various acupuncture sites.

Meditation

Meditation works; that is without a doubt. It works by rewiring the brain and increasing the volume of brain tissue in certain areas, and a simple meditation practice can transform nearly every area of your life. You don't have to be meditating for hours at a time to gain benefits. You can start with a simple 2–3 minute practice, and then extend your practice for longer periods.

Among known benefits of meditation are that it reduces stress and anxiety, improves focus, helps overcome addiction, and strengthens the immune system.

Meditation is a practice. It will continue to grow and evolve as you put more time into it. There is no end destination to meditation, and it is perfectly okay if your thoughts wander or if you lose focus. Just bring yourself back to your centre, or refocus in a gentle way. There is no competition or judgement. You are not meant to compete against another in terms of how much time you put into it or how deeply focused you are. Meditation is for you and for you alone, although the clarity and peace of mind that you get to enjoy may benefit the people around you too.

Final Thoughts on Alternative Healing

Alternative healing remedies are natural and non-invasive. They support the body's own healing processes, and rather than focusing on a specific illness or set of symptoms, they encompass a holistic approach by considering the person's mind, body, spirit, and emotions in treatment. There are many alternative healing modalities; many of them complement each other. You can meditate, have acupuncture, and take homeopathic remedies without contra-indications.

More importantly, alternative remedies are coming out of the cold and are increasingly being used in combination with conventional Western medicine, giving rise to "integrative medicine." My advice is that when it comes to your health, stay open to possibilities to find what works best for you.

**To contact Veronica Rudan,
please go to
www.drugstodistanthealing.com**

Printed in Great Britain
by Amazon

78152599R00078